PRACTICAL HANDBOOK

MASSAGE, AROMATHERAPY & YOGA

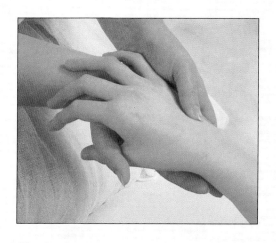

CAROLE McGILVERY, JIMI REED, MIRA MEHTA

SELECT
EDITIONS

Select Editions imprint specially produced for Selectabook Ltd.

© Anness Publishing Limited 1993, 1999

Produced by Anness Publishing Limited
Hermes House, 88-89 Blackfriars Road, London SE1 8HA

The publishers recognize Mira Mehta to be the originator
of the yoga section of this volume (pages 170-255).

ISBN 1-84081-248-6

Publisher: Joanna Lorenz
Project Editor: Elaine Collins
Photographic Assistant: Kirsty Wilson
Designer: Kit Johnson
Additional layouts: David Rowley, Lillian Lindblom
and Ian Sandom
Jacket design: Balley Design Associates
Artwork: Raymond Turvey, King & King
Illustrations on pages 162 and 163 by Michael Shoebridge

Also published as
The Encyclopedia of Aromatherapy, Massage and Yoga

Typeset by Dorchester Typesetting Group Ltd

Printed and bound in Hong Kong

1 3 5 7 9 10 8 6 4 2

ACKNOWLEDGEMENTS

The authors and publishers would like to thank the following for
their valuable contributions to the book:

Nina Ashby, Andrea Ashley, Richard Good, Angela Inverso,
Clive Ives, BKS Iyengar, Kay Kiernan, Lisa Myhill, Rachel
Stewart, Eve Taylor, Karin Weisensel and Janice Welch for advice
and contributions to the text.

Michaeljohn, The Bluestone Clinic, The Iyengar Yoga Institute,
Clarins, The Ragdale Clinic, Henlow Grange and Grayshott Hall
for providing advice, expertise and personnel.

Avalon Aromatic Candles, The Body Shop, Boutique Descampes,
Clarins, Cosmetics to Go, Culpeper, Decleor Ltd, Futon,
Gore Booker, Knickerbox, Kobashi, Nice Irma's,
Pineapple Dance Studio and Purves and Purves
for providing equipment, clothes and products.

Juliet Algie, Andrea Ashley, Mary Atkinson, Alison Barry,
Nichola Clare, Paula Clark, Laura Cream, Max Collins Wolff,
Karen Flynn, Richard Good, Eric Haines, Angela Inverso,
Clive Ives, Tabitha Jackson, Maya Jacobson, Maria Johnson,
Colette Keogh, Kerry Le Surf, Sophie Marks, Mira Mehta,
Lisa Myhill, Maria Nuccio, Sue Paterson-Jones, Anna Rand,
Glenys Shepherd, Rachel Stewart, Michelle Thomas,
David Tierney, Ormond Uren, Karin Weisensel, Janice Welch and
Karen Wilding for appearing in the photographs.

PICTURE CREDITS

The Bridgeman Art Library: p.8 top and below.
Picturepoint Limited: pp.9 and 10-11.
French Picture Library: p.11, inset below.
The Ancient Art and Architecture Collection: pp.11, inset top,
100 and 101.
Gerry Clist Photography: pp.172 and 173.

PRACTICAL HANDBOOK

MASSAGE, AROMATHERAPY & YOGA

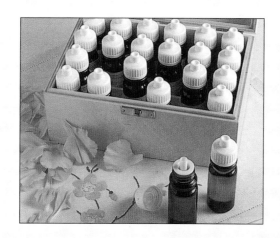

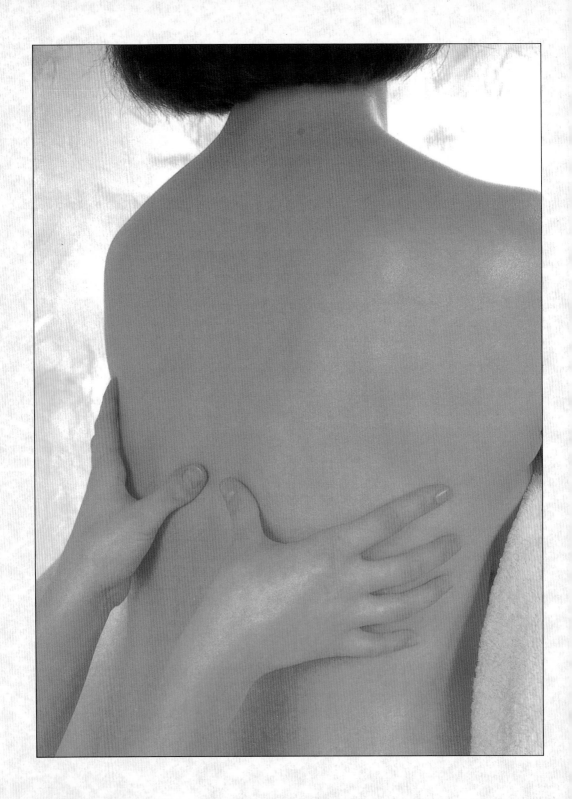

CONTENTS

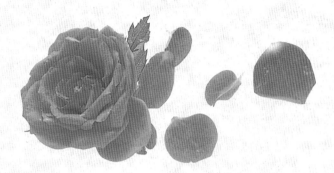

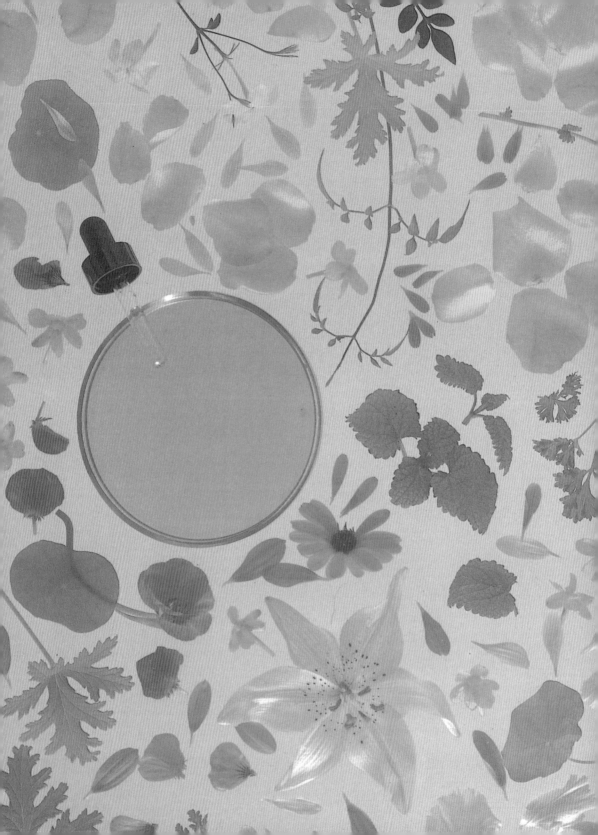

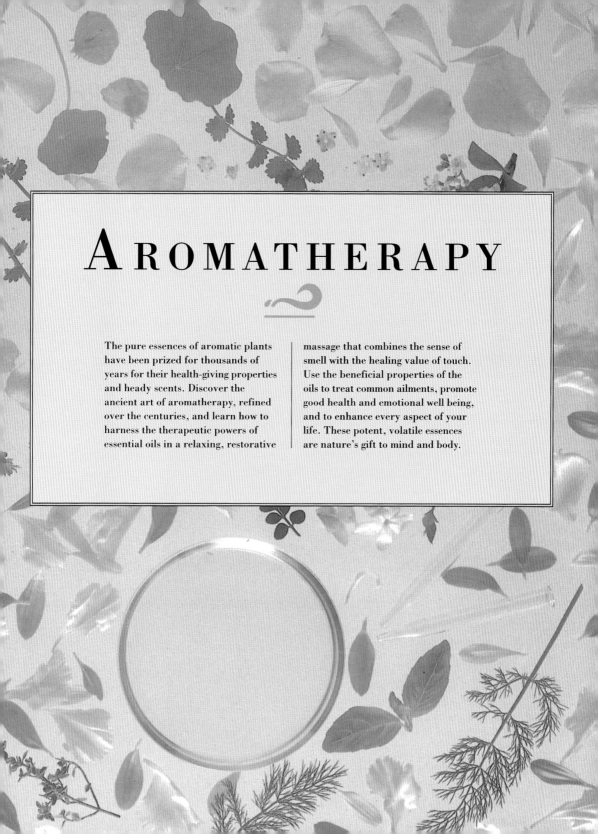

AROMATHERAPY

The pure essences of aromatic plants have been prized for thousands of years for their health-giving properties and heady scents. Discover the ancient art of aromatherapy, refined over the centuries, and learn how to harness the therapeutic powers of essential oils in a relaxing, restorative massage that combines the sense of smell with the healing value of touch. Use the beneficial properties of the oils to treat common ailments, promote good health and emotional well being, and to enhance every aspect of your life. These potent, volatile essences are nature's gift to mind and body.

AN ANCIENT ART

The value of natural plant oils has been recognized for more than 6000 years, for their healing, cleansing, preservative and mood-enhancing properties, as well as for the sheer pleasure of their fragrances. Today, these properties are being rediscovered as we look to the wisdom of past eras and civilizations to restore the balance that has been lost in modern-day life. Stress, pollution, unhealthy diet, hectic but sedentary lifestyles – all these factors have adverse effects on our bodies and spirits. The art of aromatherapy harnesses the potent pure essences of aromatic plants, flowers and resins, to work on the most powerful of senses – smell and touch – to restore the harmony of body and mind.

SECRETS OF THE OILS DISCOVERED

The origins of aromatherapy can be traced through the religious, medical and social practices of all the major civilizations. It is likely that the Chinese were the first to discover the remarkable medicinal powers of plants around 4500 BC. However, it is the Egyptians who must take the credit for recognizing and fully exploiting the physical and spiritual properties of aromatic essences. From hieroglyphs and paintings we know that aromatic preparations were used as offerings to the gods. Furthermore the natural antiseptic and antibacterial properties of essential oils and resins, particularly cedarwood and frankincense, made them ideal for the purpose of preserving corpses in preparation for the next world. The discovery of remarkably well-preserved mummies up to 5000 years after their preparation is a tribute to the embalmer's art.

By around 3000 BC priests who had been using the oils in religious ceremonies and embalming rites became aware of the usefulness of their properties for the living, too. Closely guarding their secrets, they became the healers of their time, mixing and prescribing "magic" medicinal potions. Use of essential oils gradually permeated all levels of society as cosmetics and perfumes became widespread.

From Hippocrates we know the Greeks had some awareness of the therapeutic properties of the oils and their value as sedatives and stimulants was certainly recognized. The Greeks and Romans used aromatics widely in rituals and ceremonies and the oils played an important role in the rise in popularity of baths and massage and body-culture generally. However, with the fall of the Roman Empire the use of essential oils died out in Europe.

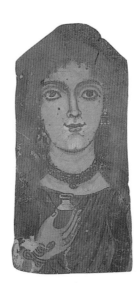

Left: The personal use of perfume was widespread in ancient Greece and Rome. The Roman girl in this portrait (from around AD 350) carries a small pot of aromatics.

Right: From the tomb of the Noble Senedjem, ancient Egypt. The cones of unguent worn on the heads melted in the heat, waxing and scenting the hair and body.

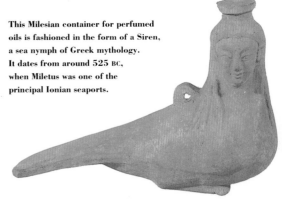

This Milesian container for perfumed oils is fashioned in the form of a Siren, a sea nymph of Greek mythology. It dates from around 525 BC, when Miletus was one of the principal Ionian seaports.

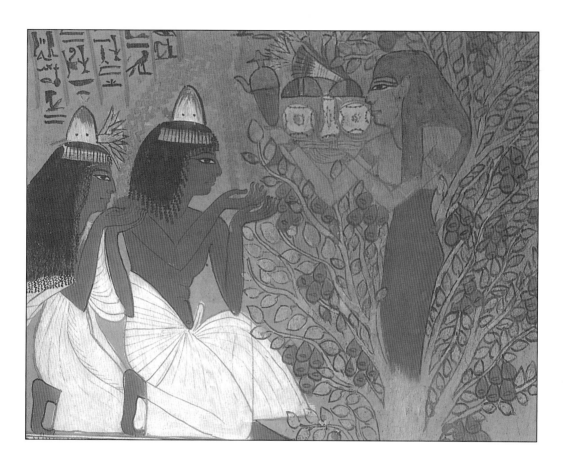

The art flourished elsewhere, though, particularly in Arabia, where Avicenna was the first to distill rose essence around AD 1000. Arabia became the world's centre for production of perfume, importing raw materials from Egypt, India, Tibet and China, and trading their products internationally.

With the Crusaders the art of perfumery was reintroduced to Europe around the twelfth century. Records show that aromatics were used as protection against the plague and the lower incidence of death among perfumiers suggests they were to some degree effective. The fifteenth century saw the rise of the great European perfumiers, and their wares were widely used to disguise body smells and ward off sickness. By the seventeenth century the aphrodisiac properties were certainly well recognized, and with the work of the great herbalists, such as Culpeper, the therapeutic properties also started to be recorded, laying the foundation for modern-day aromatherapy.

THE MODERN RENAISSANCE

The term "Aromathérapie" was first used in 1928 by a French chemist, René-Maurice Gattefossé, to describe the therapeutic action of aromatic plant essences. His work was taken up by Dr Jean Valnet who found the essences' remarkable regenerative and antiseptic properties effective for healing the wounds of World War II soldiers.

The application of aromatherapy to beauty therapy and health care was pioneered by Marguerite Maury in her influential book, *The Secret of Life and Youth*. She also developed the method of applying the oils through massage.

Today there is a world-wide revival in the art of aromatherapy and contemporary research is beginning to understand the scientific foundations of the oils' properties and applications, discovered by trial and error over thousands of years.

ESSENTIAL OILS

The vital element in any aromatherapy treatment is the pure essential oil. These oils are very different from the heavy oils we use for cooking; they are concentrated essences, much lighter than water and highly flammable. They evaporate quickly, so they are usually mixed with other ingredients to trap their effectiveness. Because they are so concentrated, essential oils are measured in drops.

ESSENCE

This is a natural living substance: the "living" element of a plant which is captured and capsuled. It is a delicate operation. For instance, certain petals and leaves must be picked at exactly the right moment, or the quality of the oil is affected. Only the purest essences are used in aromatherapy so that the therapeutic properties are maximized and the effects are predictable.

Essential oils are extracted from an array of plant sources – petals, leaves, seeds, nut kernels, bark, stalks, flower heads and gums and resins from trees. Apart from their sensuous vapours, which provide the fragrance in many perfumes, they can be used in the bath, smoothed over the body, and used in the myriad ways described in this book.

Because of their small molecular structure, essential oils can penetrate the skin more effectively than vegetable oils, which only lie on the surface. Used medicinally over the centuries, essential oils have now become an established "alternative" natural therapy which can assist in the treatment of almost every type of ache and pain, as well as smoothing away the stress and strains of modern life.

HOW THEY WORK

Essential oils are composed of tiny molecules which are easily dissolved in alcohol, emulsifiers and, particularly, fats. This allows them to penetrate the skin easily and work into the body by mixing with the fatty tissue.

As these highly volatile essences evaporate they are also inhaled, thus entering the body via the millions of sensitive cells that line the nasal passages. These send messages straight to the brain, and affect the emotions by working on the limbic system, which also controls the major functions of the body. Thus in an aromatherapy treatment the essential oils are able to enhance both your physical and psychological well-being at the same time.

Each oil has a distinct chemical composition which determines its fragrance, colour, volatility and, of course, the ways in which it affects the system, giving each oil its unique set of beneficial properties.

METHODS OF EXTRACTION

Distillation
The Egyptians stored their raw materials in large clay or alabaster pots. Water was added and the pots

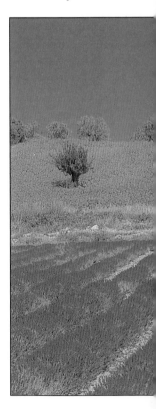

Main picture: Field of lavender, Drome, southern France. French lavender produces the finest quality oil, with a fruitier and sweeter aroma than English lavender, which has a camphorous undertone. It takes one ton (one tonne) of plants to yield about 20 lb (9 kg) of essential oil.

Inset top: Egyptian relief showing perfume-making, from the fourth century BC. The large alabaster pot (a "linge") was filled with flowers, herbs and water, and then heated. The aromatic vapours would saturate a cloth stretched across the pot's opening.

Inset below: Art meets science in the skills of the perfumier, blending a subtle new fragrance from the hundreds of essential oils at his disposal.

heated so that steam rose and was pushed through a cotton cloth in the neck of the jar. This soaked up the essential oil which was then squeezed and pressed out into a collection vessel. The same principle remains in use today as high-pressure steam is passed over the leaves or flowers in a sophisticated still often using a vacuum, so that the essential oils within them vaporize. When the steam carrying the essential oil passes through a cooling system, the oil condenses and can be separated easily from the water.

Maceration

Flowers are soaked in hot oil to break down the cells, releasing their fragrance into the oil which is then purified and the aromatics extracted.

Enfleurage

This is the method by which flower essences, such as jasmine, neroli and rose, which are more delicate and difficult to obtain, are extracted. Flowers or petals are crushed between wooden-framed, glass trays smeared with a greasy animal fat until the fat is saturated with their perfume.

Pressing

This is a simple method of squeezing out, literally, essential oils from the rinds and peel of ripe fruit, such as orange and lemon, into a sponge.

QUALITY CONTROL

Once the flowers and plants are harvested they are usually processed and stored quickly to preserve the freshness. Climate, soil and altitude can all affect the character of an oil. French lavender, for example, is famous for its rich aroma but, like wine, the quality can vary from year to year.

Always buy pure and natural essential oils as synthetic clones or adulterated oils do not act on the body in the same way and many of the beneficial properties are lost. The best quality oils may be expensive but they are always worth the extra cost.

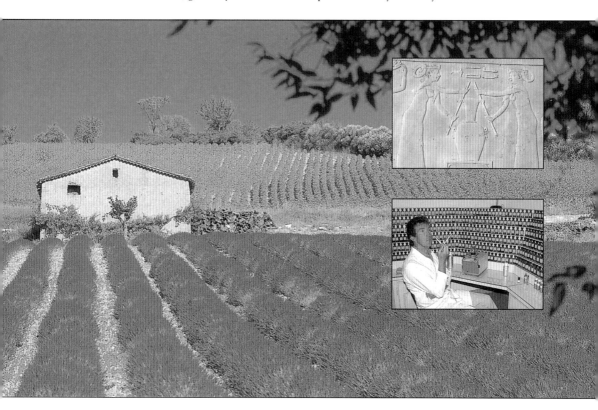

USING ESSENTIAL OILS

You can soak and splash in them, feed your skin, sensually smooth them all over, or simply breathe in their wonderful aromas. The pleasure and versatility of aromatic oils make them one of nature's kindest gifts. Essential oils contain the active ingredients of a plant in a highly concentrated and potent form. They therefore need to be treated with care and should never be applied directly to the skin undiluted. However, there are many ways of dispersing their fragrance and utilizing their therapeutic properties, and most methods do not require any special equipment.

Inhalation

Steam inhalation is an excellent method for treating respiratory problems, colds and so forth, but should not be used by asthmatics. Add 6–12 drops to a bowl of steaming hot water. Place a towel over your head and breathe deeply. This is also a great way of deep-cleansing the face.

Therapeutic Massage

This is the classic aromatherapy treatment, triggering the body's natural healing process by using lymphatic massage and essential oils to stimulate the flow of blood and lymph fluid. The aromas also act upon the emotional centre in the brain (the "limbic" system) which governs the way we feel.

For massage use a 1–3 per cent solution of essential oil to base oil.

Fragrancers

These attractive pots, also known as diffusers or vaporizers, are simple to use. Fill the top china bowl with water and add a few drops of essential oil on to the surface. The candle in the pot underneath heats the water, slowly releasing the natural fragrance of the oil into the room.

Stand the burner on a plate or tile, not on plastic surfaces.

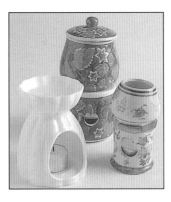

Decorative fragancers for diffusing essential oils.

3–6 drops of essential oil are sufficient, depending on the size of the room. It is also possible to buy battery-driven fan vaporizers which blow air through oil-impregnated pads, which can be changed to suit the mood.

Baths

Run hand-hot water and then add 5–10 drops of the essential oil to suit your mood. Close the door, keep in the vapours, and soak for 15 minutes. For sensitive skin it is better to dilute the oil in a base oil first, like sweet almond, apricot or peach kernel. Essential oils can mark plastic baths if they are not dispersed thoroughly. Wipe the bath straight after use.

Foot Bath

Refresh tired feet by adding 4–5 drops of peppermint, rosemary and thyme to a large bowl of hot water. Soothe with lavender.

Hand Bath

Soothe chapped skin by soaking in bowl of warm water (not hot) with 3–4 drops of patchouli or comfrey before a manicure.

Shower

After soaping or gelling, rinse well. Dip a wet sponge in an oil mix of your choice, squeeze and rub over your whole body while under a warm jet spray.

Sauna

Add two drops of eucalyptus or pine oil per $\frac{1}{2}$ pint (330 ml) of water and throw over the coals to evaporate. These are great cleansers and detoxifiers.

Jacuzzi or Hot Tub

Relax by adding 10–15 drops of sandalwood, geranium or ylang-ylang, or simply bubble over with the stimulating effects of pine, rosemary and neroli.

Room Sprays

To make a room spray blend ten drops of essential oil in seven tablespoons of water. One tablespoon of vodka or pure alcohol added to the solution will act as a preservative but this is optional. Shake well before filling the sprayer.

Pillow Talk

Perfume your pillow with 2–3 drops of oil. Choose a relaxing oil to unwind or one for insomnia if you have sleep problems. For a different mood, try an aphrodisiac like ylang-ylang or be extravagant and use rose or jasmine, the two most expensive pure oils.

Perfumes

The finest perfumes are traditionally blended from pure essential oils, particularly the flower extracts, though these days synthetic aromas tend to be used, particularly for cheaper perfumes. The art of the perfumier is subtle and skilled, and difficult to emulate at home as it is hard to find a medium to use as a substitute for alcohol. If you have a favourite oil or blend of essences you can use it all over in a body oil (three per cent solution), or make a very concentrated blend (25 per cent) to dab behind ears, knees and on wrists and temples.

Pomanders

Hang porous corked bottles in the wardrobe. The essential oil is absorbed by the clay and released slowly. Fill with the fragrance of your choice: try melissa or bergamot, or cedarwood to keep away moths.

Pot Pourri

Add a few drops of an appropriate flowery or spicy essential oil to refresh tired pot pourri, or make your own.

Handkerchief

The most portable way of using essential oils. Add 3–4 drops to a handkerchief and inhale. Useful for treating colds or headaches, or for clearing your head at work.

Shoe Rack

Freshen the cupboard with lemongrass. Deodorize shoes with two drops of pine or parsley oil.

From the top: perfume bottle, pot pourri and oil lamp.

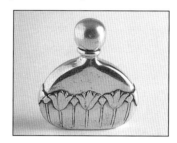

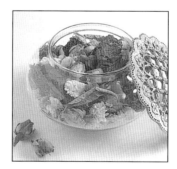

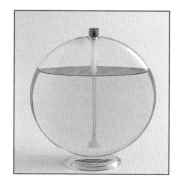

Humidifiers

You can add your favourite oil to the water of a humidifier or improvize by adding five drops of essential oil to a small bowl of water placed on top of a radiator.

Ring Burners

Use the heat from light bulbs to release perfumed oils. Small ring burners, usually made of porcelain or aluminium, sit over the top of the bulb. Add a few drops of essential oil, and the heat from the bulb will gently vaporize the essential oil.

Wood Fires

Sprinkle drops of cypress, cedarwood, pine or sandalwood over the logs to be used about an hour before lighting the fire and then burn them to release your favourite aroma.

Scented Candles

Wax candles can be bought ready-impregnated with essential oils and are a delightful way of fragrancing a room. Or you can add a few drops of essential oil to an oil lamp for the same effect.

Compresses

Soak a clean cotton cloth (such as a face flannel, handkerchief or small towel) in $\frac{1}{4}$ pint (160 ml) warm water with 5–10 drops of essential oil. Squeeze out and lay across the area to be treated. Cover and leave until cold. A useful method for sprains, bruising, headaches (place the compress across the forehead) and hot flushes.

Body and Facial Oils

These can be used on a daily basis to nourish the skin. Use a one per cent blend of essential oil to carrier oil for the face and a three per cent blend for the body.

BLENDING AND STORING

Essential oils are the basis for all traditional Aromatherapy. Each one has a particular fragrance and properties and the art of blending them harmoniously combines the skills of the perfumier and the pharmacist. Although two essences may have a similar smell or property they may not necessarily mix well together. One essence can overpower the other. For example, frankincense and ginger, both heavy smelling essences, give an overpowering, unpleasant smell when combined, whereas lavender and rosemary happily marry together. In general it is best to use a maximum of three oils in a blend so there is less chance of detracting from their individual qualities.

Assemble bottles of different sizes for storing appropriate quantities of blended oils. Funnels and droppers ensure accurate measurements and help prevent spillages.

THE ART OF BLENDING

Essential oils are highly volatile substances which should be handled, mixed and stored with care and used sparingly. Spillage of one particular oil can overpower a whole room and adversely affect young children and animals.

The power of aromatics is quite subtle. Never try to sniff or smell a pure essential oil straight from the bottle. Place a drop on the side of a glass and become a connoisseur: sniff, consider and take notes if you wish.

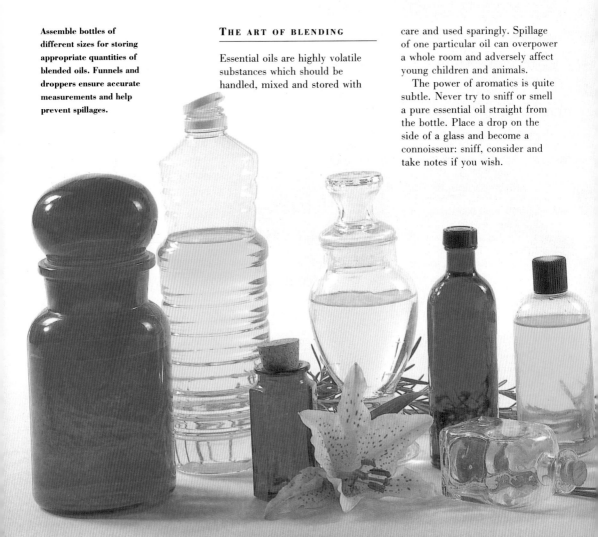

MIXING

Base oils play an important role in carrying and diluting highly concentrated essential oils, which are only used in small quantities measured in drops. These base oils dilute the pure essentials, inhibiting the evaporation rate and – since they spread evenly and easily over skin – encouraging quick absorption of the therapeutic oils into the skin.

When mixing, use a glass, porcelain or aluminium bottle and check that you have the correct amount of vegetable carrier oil before adding the recommended drops of essentials with a dropper or pipette for accurate measurements. Mix well and label the bottles clearly.

If you accidentally spill any, wipe up instantly with a paper tissue and dispose of it outside as the smell will be overpowering.

STORING

Dark glass bottles with stoppered caps are used to store essential oils. At home, keep them in a cool dark place, stand them upright, and always out of sight and touch of children. Never store essential oils in plastic bottles: both the oil and the bottle will perish. Oils will keep for at least a year if properly stored, although citrus oils may have a shorter life.

CARRIER OILS

ase oils are normally extracted from nuts or seeds and each has its own particular quality. Sweet almond oil is probably the best all-purpose carrier oil because it is neutral and non-allergenic. It can even be used for massaging babies. Walnut acts as a co-ordinator and balances the nervous system; sesame is ideal for stretch marks; apricot kernel, peach kernel and evening primrose oils are all good for cell regeneration. Walnut and evening primrose oil help alleviate menstrual problems including pre-menstrual tension. Wheatgerm acts as an anti-oxidant and will help preserve a mixture.

These oils are all rich in nutrients, and are ideal for most dry and sensitive skin types. The most important thing when buying these basics is to check that they have been naturally processed and not chemically treated. Cold-pressed is best.

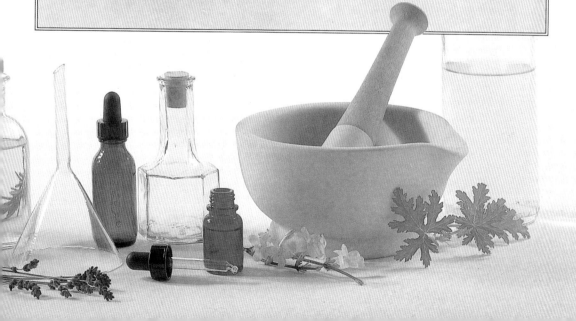

AROMATICS

Aromatic oils extracted from flowers, fruits, leaves, barks, resins and roots have been used throughout the centuries for their healing properties and marvellous fragrances. Hundreds of essential oils are used today in such industries as food, cosmetics, pharmaceuticals and perfumery. Modern-day aromatherapy uses a much smaller selection, but the range of aromas and applications is nonetheless remarkable.

This section is a connoisseurs' guide to thirty-five of the most popular, versatile and safe oils. Get to know their individual characters, their origins, their therapeutic values and discover your own favourites. Lavender, geranium and rosemary are excellent all-round oils and provide a good basis for any collection. Rose, though expensive, is also well worth the investment if you would like to explore the benefits and delights of aromatherapy.

BASIL

Ocimum basilicum

Origins Basil was used in baths and body massage by ancient Greek nobles for its fragrant perfume. The Egyptians used the aromatic fragrance in their offerings to the gods and also mixed it with essences of myrrh and incense to embalm bodies. In India it is believed to offer protection to the soul and is sacred to the Hindu gods Krishna and Vishnu.

Description Native of Africa and the Seychelles and now grown as a popular culinary herb in Europe, it can grow up to three feet (90 cm) in height and has small white flowers. The essence is distilled from the leaves and is a light greenish-yellow with sweet green overtones.

Therapeutic effects Ideal as a nerve tonic, to lift fatigue, anxiety and depression. Also good for bronchitis, colds, fever, gout and indigestion, and reputed to soothe snake bites.

Uses Inhalation, baths and massage. It has both hot and cold qualities. When used in the bath or smoothed over the body it has an invigorating effect – great for sluggish skin and pepping up circulation. Combined with other oils such as thyme it also acts as a powerful antiseptic.

Cautionary note A powerful depressant if over-used. Also best to avoid during pregnancy.

BAY

Pimenta racemosa

Origins Roman emperors wore sprigs of bay, known as *Laurus nobilis* (Roman laurel), not only as a sign of wealth, but to ward off evil spirits. Greek priestesses chewed the leaves for their soporific effect, and after gastronomic banquets it was chewed as a breath freshener.

Description Popular as a culinary herb, bay is an attractive evergreen shrub whose shiny leathery leaves produce clusters of yellowish-green flowers in spring. The spicy-smelling oil is extracted from the leaves and is yellowish-brown in colour.

Therapeutic effects As a pulmonary antiseptic, it helps relieve bronchitis, colds and flu. Also used to aid digestion and sleep, to soothe rheumatic aches and pains, and as a general tonic.

Uses Inhalation, baths and massage. Widely used in perfume and exotic bath essences for its uplifting effects.

BENZOIN

Styrax benzoin

Origins In the Far East the gum from the benzoin tree was one of the main ingredients used in incense to drive away evil spirits. The compound tincture is highly potent, pharmaceutically used in friar's balsam and as a fixative in perfume.

Description The benzoin tree is cultivated in Borneo, Java, Malaysia, Sumatra and Thailand. Like the rubber tree, its gum is taken from the bark by making a deep incision in the trunk. The gum is dark, with reddish-brown coloured streaks. These pigments contain the fatty oils which exude a delicious aroma similar to vanilla.

Therapeutic effects Valuable for treating urinary infections, it has a warming, relaxing, action suitable for respiratory conditions such as bronchitis, coughs and colds. Also effective for relieving skin conditions, and for gout.

Uses Inhalation, massage and in cough medicines. This is an energizing oil which can be used in one of two forms: simple tincture or compound – the former is not so toxic and is preferable for skin conditions.

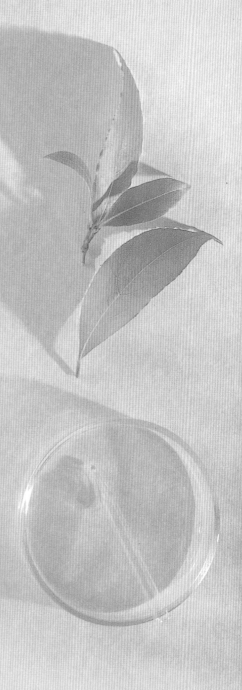

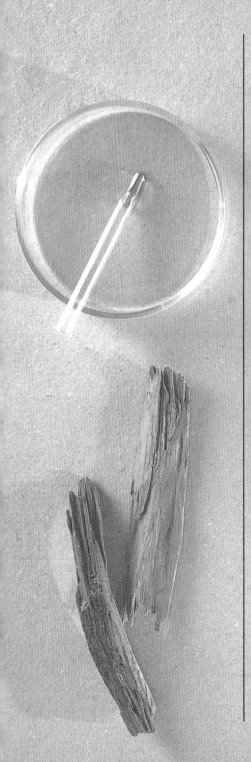

BERGAMOT
Citrus bergamia

Origins Native to Morocco, it wasn't until bergamot rooted in Italy that its essential properties were recognized.

Description The bergamot tree belongs to the same family as the orange tree and the essential oil, as in most citrus varieties, is expressed from the fresh peel of the fruit. The oil is emerald green in colour, and smells spicier than lemon but with a similar, citrus quality. The odour is familiar from its use as a flavouring in Earl Grey tea.

Therapeutic effects Has a powerful uplifting and refreshing action. As an antiseptic it has proved effective in the treatment of mouth and skin infections, and sore throats. Can lower fever, and help with bronchitis and indigestion.

Uses Bergamot blends well with most essences and is a popular top note in perfumery. Along with neroli and lavender it is a main ingredient in eau-de-Cologne and is commonly used in toiletries to refresh and relax. In massage it can stimulate or soothe depending on the oils with which it is mixed.

Cautionary note In concentrations above one per cent it can irritate the skin. Also, even though it is sometimes added to commercial suntan agents to stimulate melanin production, it must never be used in home mixtures for tanning purposes.

CEDARWOOD
Juniperus virginiana

Origins Cedarwood oil, similar to sandalwood, was used by the Egyptians in the embalming process. It was highly prized for its antiseptic properties and so became an important ingredient in cosmetics. Originally it was made from the beautiful Lebanon cedar, but, over-felled for furniture, this is now very scarce, and the red cedar is primarily used in its place.

Description The cedar is grown in North Africa and the USA for its highly valued, fragrant wood. The clear, syrupy essential oil is extracted by steam distillation of waste woods. The odour of the oil is reminiscent of wooden pencils.

Therapeutic effects Used for skin complaints such as acne, alopecia, dandruff and eczema, and respiratory problems, especially bronchitis and catarrh. Also acts as a diuretic for help in urinary infections.

Uses Inhalation and massage. Increases sexual response. Blends well with cypress, juniper and rose.

Cautionary note Will irritate the skin in high concentrations.

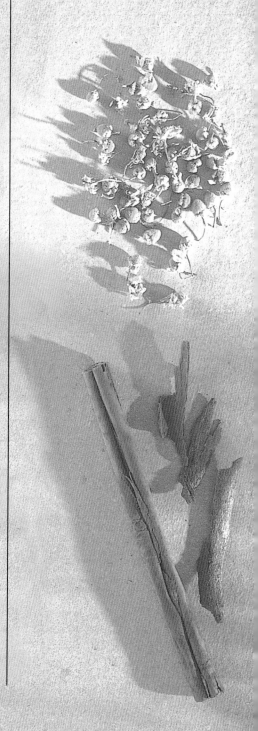

CHAMOMILE
Alternative spelling: Camomile

Anthemis nobilis

Origins The Egyptians thought this was a sacred flower and dedicated it to the Sun God. It was used in ritual ceremonies and medicinally to stop fits and fevers.

Description Chamomile species grow throughout Europe, North Africa and are often found growing wild. They have fine, feathery leaves with tiny white or yellow-centred daisy-like flowers. The pale blue oil is extracted from the flower and has a slightly apple fragrance which blends well with rose, geranium and lavender.

Therapeutic effects Particularly noted for its anti-inflammatory and sedative properties, it is excellent for childhood ailments (whether in children or adults!) from peevishness to earache. Also used for allergies, anaemia, burns, dermatitis, diarrhoea, fever, indigestion, insomnia, menstrual and menopausal problems, rheumatism, toothache and ulcers.

Uses Certain chamomile species are used for herbal infusions, but the oil is used in body, bath and hair products for its anti-allergenic properties. Use in dilute form for children.

CINNAMON

Cinnamomum zeylanicum

Origins The Chinese believed that no remedy or treatment was complete without cinnamon. It is one of the oldest spices known – used by the Egyptians, Romans and Greeks, and it was also mentioned in the Old Testament.

Description Grown in the Far East, East Indies, and China, cinnamon has a distinctive hot, peppery aroma and taste. The twigs and leaves are picked and distilled to produce a sweet, pungent and bitter aromatic oil, which is a dark yellow-brown in colour. Its warm, spicy essence is often used in perfumery.

Therapeutic effects Useful for fatigue and depression, it is also a tonic for the respiratory and digestive systems, especially useful for coughs, colds, flu, stomach ache and diarrhoea. An aphrodisiac, it may also help impotence.

Uses Inhalation and massage. Burn to prevent the spread of flu virus, or add bark or oil to spice up a pot pourri. To relieve muscular spasms use in a compress or massage.

Cautionary note Use only in very low concentrations or under professional advice.

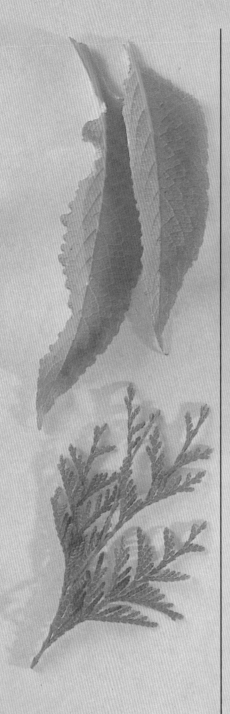

COMFREY

Symphtum officinale

Origins Herbalist Nicholas Culpeper wrote in his medicinal scripts in the seventeenth century that this herb 'helpeth those that spit blood or make a bloody urine'. The root boiled in water or wine was drunk to help solve all internal problems, inwardly healing wounds, ulcers of the lungs and to help the flow of blood.

Description Normally grows wild near damp watersides. Comfrey has large hairy leaves which can irritate the skin if touched. The stalk grows to three feet (90 cm) high with pale purplish flowers. The leaves and roots are used in herbal decoctions but the oil is extracted from the leaves and stalks.

Therapeutic effects Containing allantoin, a cell regenerator, comfrey oil is particularly valuable for the treatment of wounds and skin disorders, including eczema, psoriasis, athlete's foot and torn muscles. Helpful, too, in treating stretch marks and for menopausal and menstrual problems.

Uses Massage and compresses.

CYPRESS

Cupressus sempervirens

Origins Egyptians used this wood to adorn their stone coffins along with using the oil for its medicinal properties. In France it is traditionally planted in graveyards.

Description A tall, conical, evergreen tree, it originated in the East but is popularly grown throughout the Mediterranean area, especially in Algeria and southern France. The essence is obtained by the distillation of the leaves, twigs and cones of the tree. Clear, pale yellow or green, it has a refreshing, spicy fragrance, reminiscent of pine-needles.

Therapeutic effects Most noted for its astringent and antispasmodic qualities, it can be used for circulatory conditions, colds, coughs, flu, haemorrhoids, menstrual and menopausal problems, varicose veins and whooping cough. It also acts as a sedative to soothe nervous tension.

Uses Inhalation, baths and massage. Use in compresses for swelling or rheumatism or in the bath as a muscular tonic. Its astringent properties make it suitable for use in cleansers for oily skin.

Cautionary note Not to be used by anyone who suffers from high blood pressure.

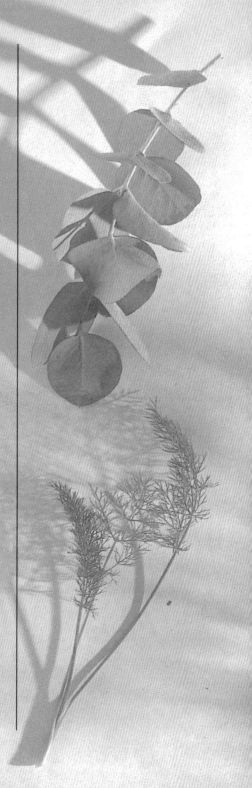

EUCALYPTUS
Eucalyptus globulus

Origins One of the tallest trees in the world, it originated in Australia and later grew in Tasmania, China, USA, Brazil and the Mediterranean. There are something like 200 species. The Aborigines may have been the first to use it medicinally.

Description The silvery, blue–green leaves produce a pale yellow oil which has a cool, camphorous smell. The fresh leaves give a rich yield of highly potent essence, one of the most versatile in aromatherapy.

Therapeutic effects The principal constituent of the oil is the antiseptic eucalyptol. Combined with its anti-inflammatory properties, eucalyptus oil is particularly helpful for asthma, bronchitis, flu, sinusitis, skin infections, rheumatism and sores. It can also reduce fever, is a strong diuretic, and its head-clearing qualities are well-known.

Uses Baths, inhalation and massage. It has a cooling effect on body temperature, reduces fever and is also a remedy for muscular/rheumatic aches and pains. It is widely used in cold and cough medicines and rubs. Use in the bath to relieve cystitis or on a handkerchief to clear the head.

FENNEL
Foeniculum vulgare

Origins The ancient Greeks and Romans advocated the strongly flavoured fennel seeds to give them strength, to ward off evil spirits, kill fleas, and sweeten the breath.

Description These graceful perennial plants are found in Europe, often by the sea, and have delicate bright green feathery foliage. Their bright tufts of yellow flowers attract the bees. As a herb, the fresh leaves are particularly valued for fish dishes whereas the seeds, which smell like aniseed, are used in liquorice. The sweet oil, which has a similar smell, is extracted from the crushed seeds.

Therapeutic effects Noted as a diuretic, and a mild laxative, fennel has been found effective for colic, constipation, digestive problems, kidney stones, menopausal problems, nausea and obesity. It is also often helpful for increasing milk yield during breast feeding.

Uses Massage. The sweet aromatic oil is mainly used for flavouring medicines to help flatulence and indigestion. It is a constituent of gripe water, and can be infused in teas.

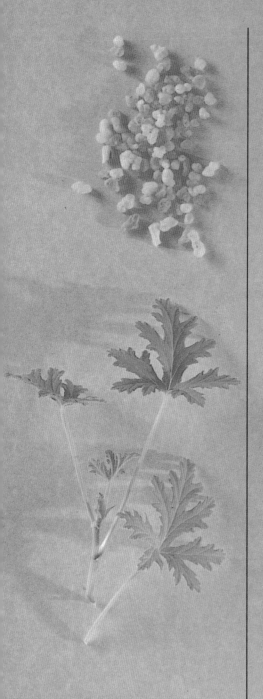

FRANKINCENSE
Boswellia thurifera

Origins Frankincense (also known as olibanum) and myrrh were the first tree resins used as incense by the Egyptians. They were burned to clear the air in sickrooms and during religious ceremonies to drive away evil spirits. They ranked alongside precious stones as a valuable commodity and, according to the Bible, were offered by the three Kings to celebrate the birth of Jesus Christ. The gum comes from a small tree grown in Arabia, Africa, and China. It was first brought to Europe in the late seventeenth century.

Description To make the gum a deep incision is made in the tree trunk where the resin exudes in tear-shaped globules which harden on contact with air. The essence is spicy, with camphor undertones, but becomes lemony when mixed with myrrh.

Therapeutic effects Has an uplifting effect and aids concentration. Helpful as an expectorant in cases of bronchitis, coughs, colds and laryngitis. Reputed to preserve a youthful skin, eradicating wrinkles.

Uses Inhalation, baths and massage. Inhale to release catarrh, or relax with a few drops in a bath or body massage oil to warm, relax and meditate. It is often combined with myrrh, and blends well with essences such as basil and sandalwood.

GERANIUM
Pelargonium adorantissimum

Origins The geranium originates in Africa and was not brought into Europe until 1690. It was used in ancient times as a remedy for tumours, burns and wounds.

Description Widely grown throughout Europe, it reaches around two feet (60 cm) in height. There are hundreds of different species cultivated for their pretty flowers, but only the aromatic pelargoniums (the ones that smell lemony when the leaves are pinched) give rich yields of the sweet yellowy-green essential oil. This is distilled from the leaves, stalks and flowers.

Therapeutic effects Unusually, it is both sedative and uplifting, and so invaluable for treating nervous tension and depression. Also used for circulatory and skin problems, especially wounds. Use in a footbath for chilblains.

Uses All uses. A popular ingredient in perfumes for its sweet, fresh, floral essence, the geranium is also therapeutically massaged or inhaled for its relaxing yet refreshing qualities. It can blend well with most other essential oils.

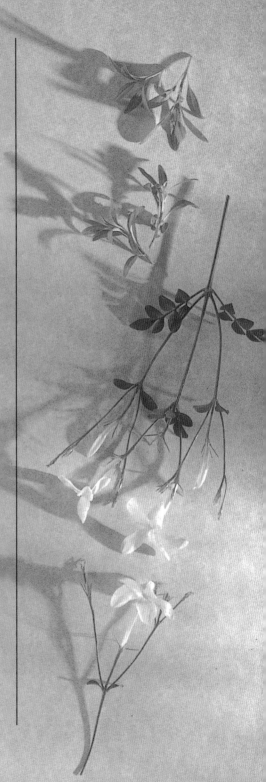

HYSSOP

Hyssopus officinalis

Origins Ancient alchemists used the powdered leaves and roots as a purgative and in ointments to spread over the stomach to combat worms. Small doses taken internally were mixed with honey to clean the mucous matter from the intestines or with crushed figs to loosen the bowels.

Description A small herbal perennial, hyssop has long stalks with narrow leaves and blue flowers. The oil, extracted from the leaves and flowering heads, is used in perfumes and liqueurs, including Chartreuse.

Therapeutic effects Hyssop is used for disorders of the cardiovascular system, and as it is both stimulating and sedative, it can regulate blood pressure whether high or low. It has powerful effects on the respiratory tract, for bronchitis, coughs and colds, and is also used for skin disorders.

Uses Massage and inhalation. It is also used in cough mixtures for bronchial conditions.

Cautionary note Use only in extremely small quantities. Do not use during pregnancy.

JASMINE

Jasminum officinale

Origins An ancient favourite of the Arabs, Indians and Chinese, jasmine had a wide variety of uses including perfuming the body, scenting rooms and flavouring herbal teas. It was introduced from Persia to Europe in the sixteenth century.

Description The *Jasminum grandiflora* species is a small bush, native to the East Indies and Egypt and cultivated in southern France, Spain, Algeria, Morocco, India and Egypt. Its delicate white flowers produce a honey-sweet floral bouquet with fruity undertones. The deep red oil is produced by *enfleurage*, and has an intense rich, floral fragrance that is warm and exotic. It is one of the most important and expensive extracts, along with rose, used in perfumery.

Therapeutic effects Jasmine is a mood enhancer, lifting anxiety and depression. An aphrodisiac, it has a reputation for the treatment of both frigidity and impotence. It will also relieve menstrual cramps and is soothing to inflamed or irritated skin.

Uses Inhalation, bathing and massage will all exploit its warming and relaxing qualities. Also makes a delightful uplifting perfume or room fragrance.

23

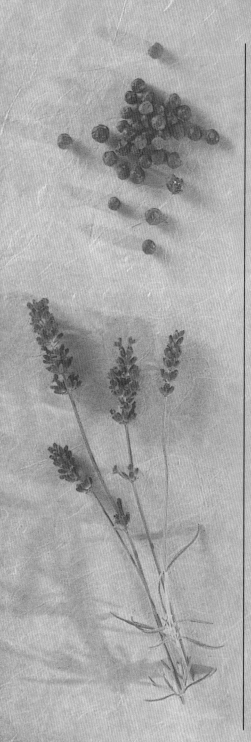

JUNIPER
Juniperus communis

Origins Grown in North America, Asia, Africa and Europe, this small shrub with aromatic leaves and berries was popular as incense to burn in religious ceremonies and to purify the air and ward off the plague.

Description An evergreen bush with thick branches and narrow needle leaves, juniper produces small yellow flowers and small purplish-blue berries. Both the berries and leaves have a strong aromatic fragrance, similar to pine-needles, but the oil is extracted from the berries by distillation, producing a pale yellow essence.

Therapeutic effects Diuretic and antiseptic, it is especially effective for the urinary tract and an excellent treatment for cystitis and water retention. Use for acne, colic, coughs, dermatitis, eczema, flatulence, rheumatism and skin ulcers.

Uses Inhalation, baths and massage. The oil is a great stimulator and, like cypress and pine, makes a refreshing bath oil. Massaged on the skin it stimulates the circulation.

LAVENDER
Lavendula officinalis

Origins Lavender comes from the Roman word "lavare" meaning to wash. It was one of most favoured aromatics used by the Romans in their daily bathing rituals. Both the Greeks and Romans burned lavender twigs as a room purifier to ward off the plague. It was brought to Europe by the Romans.

Description A shrubby plant with woody branches and long narrow leaves, it has purple-blue flowers on long spikes. After cutting, the plants are dried and steam-distilled. The essential oil is clear to pale yellow in colour with a strong aroma.

Therapeutic effects Its sedative and tonic effects make lavender a great balancer of the nervous and emotional systems. Excellent for migraine. As an antiseptic it can be used for many skin conditions and infections of the lungs, digestion and unrinary tract. Extraordinarily versatile.

Uses Inhalation, baths, room spray, massage and most other uses. Use as a cold compress or place a few drops in boiling water and inhale for headaches and migraine. A warm towel wrap will soothe nervous exhaustion. A late-night lavender bath will help combat sleeplessness.

LEMON

Citrus limonum

Origins Early seafarers stocked up with fresh lemons before a long voyage to help prevent scurvy and to purify the ship's drinking water. Its astringent and antiseptic properties were fully appreciated in the first aid kit and used to treat cuts, bruises and insect stings.

Description The lemon tree, which has white–pink flowers and bright yellow fruits, is cultivated in most Mediterranean countries, Brazil, USA, Argentina, Israel and Africa. The pale yellow oil is expressed from the rind and peel of the fruit and has classically been used in perfume for its intense, sharp, citrus-fresh aroma. The essence becomes cloudy, and deteriorates over time, if not properly stored.

Therapeutic effects Lemon is highly antiseptic and astringent, and so is naturally used for skin complaints including boils, warts and veruccas. Also good for lowering blood pressure, colds, digestive problems, fever and gallstones.

Uses Inhalation, baths and massage. Lemon, as with most citrus oils, is a good cleanser inside and out. Use in skin-care preparations for oily skin. Evaporated in a fragrancer it will help colds and act as an insect repellent.

LEMONGRASS

Cymbopogon citratus

Origins This sweet-scented grass was mainly used to season food in India, the African Congo, the Seychelles, Indonesia and Sri Lanka. Its main constituent, citral, was discovered to be a strong, cleansing antiseptic, and used to deodorize clothing and footwear. Dried leaves were burned to keep the mind alert.

Description Lemongrass is a tall-stemmed, grass-like tropical plant. Its oil is steam-distilled from the fresh or partly dried grasses, and has a refreshing, lemony smell. It is used in low-cost citrus soaps, perfumes and cleaning agents.

Therapeutic effects Through its anti-bacterial action, it is good for skin complaints, sore throats and respiratory problems. Also effective against headaches.

Uses Inhalation and massage. For the active work-out enthusiast, lemongrass is the ideal cooler and deodorizer. It can help alleviate athlete's foot and its refreshing fragrance acts as an energizer. Massaged or breathed in, it tones the heart and works on the digestive system. The oil will also repel insects.

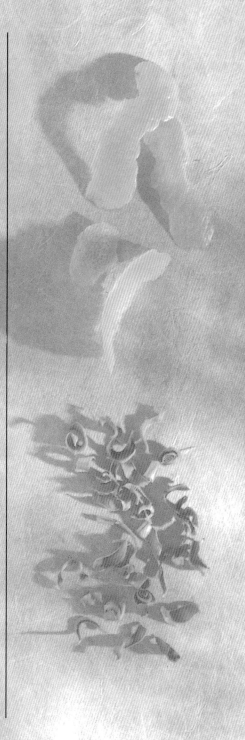

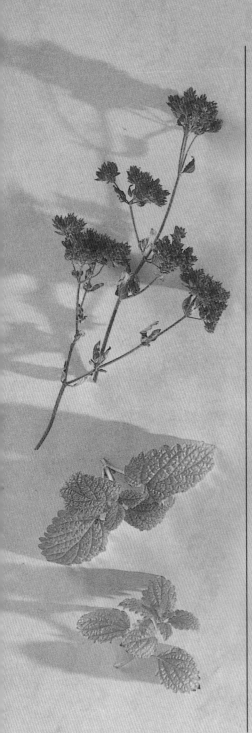

MARJORAM
Origanum marjorana

Origins The Greeks grew marjoram for use in their perfumes and herbal potions. They prescribed it as a medicinal antidote and to purge the system.

Description This popular perennial plant is one of the classic culinary herbs, and is grown world-wide. The amber-coloured essence is extracted by steam-distillation from the fresh and dried leaves and flowering tops. Its warm and slightly spicy aroma is often used in masculine fragrances.

Therapeutic effects A warming agent, able to relieve spasm, it is particularly valuable for treating the nervous system. Use for anxiety and insomnia, but also for arthritis, asthma, bronchitis, circulatory problems, constipation, headaches, menstrual problems, muscular strains and rheumatism.

Uses Inhalation and massage. It blends well with bergamot, lavender and rosemary. In bath and body oils it gives a warm, relaxing feeling. Steam-inhaled or smoothed over the sinuses and temples, it can relieve colds.

Cautionary note Do not use in early pregnancy. Do not use in high doses as it can have a narcotic effect and is also known to curb sexual drive.

MELISSA
Melissa officinalis

Origins The Greeks and Arabs knew the properties of melissa and in the sixteenth century the Swiss physician Paracelsus hailed it as the "elixir of life"

Description Mostly a native of Europe, it is also cultivated in North America. Better known as sweet balm or lemon balm, it is a bushy perennial of the mint family. The aromatic oil smells like lemons and is extracted from the leaves by distillation.

Therapeutic effects Long known as an uplifting and calming cure for "melancholia", its tonic, antispasmodic properties make it effective too in the treatment of allergies, colds, diarrhoea, hypertension, menstrual problems, migraine and stress headaches, nausea and palpitations.

Uses Inhalation, baths and massage. The essential oil helps lower blood pressure and remove tension. Add six drops to the bath water. Melissa calms the body and mind, yet lifts the soul: an oil to dream with.

MYRRH
Commiphora myrrha

Origins The Egyptians and the Greeks prized myrrh as a precious commodity. It was used by both civilizations in worshipping their gods, celebration rituals, cosmetics, perfumes and herbal treatments. The Egyptians combined it with frankincense for embalming and purification purposes.

Description A small tree, rather like a bush, myrrh is native in Arabia, Somalia, Ethiopia and other North African countries. Although the leaves are aromatic it is the resin which is distilled to produce the viscous, yellow essential oil. It has a warm, lightly spicy, sweet smell.

Therapeutic effects Anti-inflammatory and expectorant, myrrh will ease bronchitis, catarrh, coughs and colds. Good too for digestive problems, infections of the mouth and throat, and skin conditions.

Uses Inhalation and massage. It is used in pharmaceuticals and perfumery. In aromatherapy, because of its cooling effect, it blends well with camphor and lavender.

NEROLI
Citrus aurantium

Origins Neroli is believed to have been discovered by the Romans. In 1680 it was used to scent the bath water and gloves of Anna Maria Orsini, Princess of Nerola, who brought the fragrance into fashion amongst the Italian aristocracy.

Description Neroli oil is better known as orange blossom. It comes from the white blossoms of the bitter orange tree which originated in China but also grows in Egypt, Morocco, Algeria, USA, Italy and southern France. The pale yellow oil is expensive to produce since it takes approximately one ton (one tonne) of flowers to extract just 2 lb (1 kg) of oil. These are hand picked as they are just about to open and then distilled. Its powerful, wonderfully uplifting, floral fragrance is reminiscent of lilies and is extensively used in eau-de-Cologne.

Therapeutic effects An excellent sedative and anti-depressant, neroli counters anxiety, hysteria, shock and palpitations, and combats insomnia. It is helpful for dermatitis and dry skin, pre-menstrual tension and menopausal problems.

Uses Inhalation, baths and massage. Use in the bath or as a body oil to alleviate the symptoms of pre-menstrual tension and generally improve circulation, or just for the benefits of its delightful fragrance and relaxing properties.

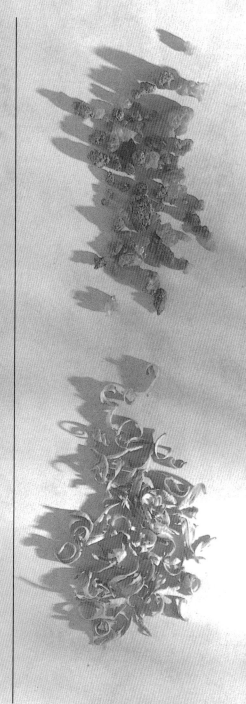

ORANGE

Citrus aurantium (bitter orange),
Citrus sinensis (sweet orange)

Origins China was the first home of the orange tree and the fragrant qualities of sweet and bitter orange oils have long been prized for culinary, cosmetic and medicinal use.

Description The sweet and the bitter oils are similar and both are extracted by cold pressing of fresh orange peel (it is only neroli oil which is extracted from the blossom). The bitter and sweet oils range from yellow to brown in colour and are used extensively for their fresh top notes in perfume.

Therapeutic effects Refreshing but sedative, orange is a tonic for anxiety and depression. It also stimulates the digestive system and is effective for constipation. Its antiseptic properties work well for mouth ulcers.

Uses Baths and massage. These essential oils, rich in vitamin C, are used widely throughout the food and cosmetics industry in products ranging from bath and body oils to chocolate-orange confectionery.

PARSLEY

Petroselinum sativum

Origins A lot of folklore surrounds the parsley plant. It was a medieval belief that it grew in the garden only if the man or woman of the house was "honest". When chewed, it would keep away the devil or, as later discovered, reduce bad breath.

Description Native to Asia Minor, it is now found all over the world. The common parsley is cultivated for its culinary uses and essential oil properties. The highest content of oil comes from the ripe seeds but the leaves are also used in distillation. It has a warm, herbaceous, spicy smell and is used in many herbal perfumes and cosmetic products.

Therapeutic effects A diuretic, useful for kidney and urinary problems and water retention. Also high in vitamin A – essential for healthy hair, skin, teeth and eyes; and iron – for the blood and liver, and during menstruation and menopause.

Uses Massage. It blends well with fennel to help combat excessive water retention when massaged over the body. In conjunction with lemon and rosemary it can help clear toxins in the liver and kidneys. In general, a good oil to help calm the nervous system.

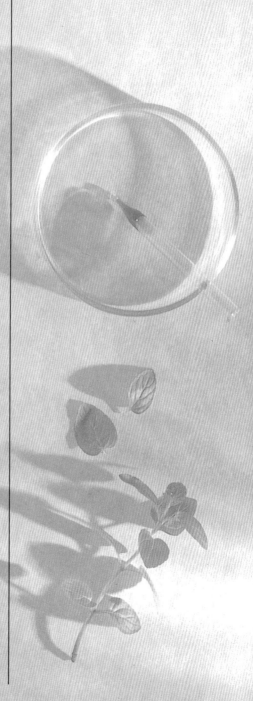

PATCHOULI
Pogostemon patchouli

Origins Along with rose, jasmine, sandalwood and basil, patchouli was one of the favourite perfumes used in India, and shawls and blankets were impregnated with this rich oil. It is an aphrodisiac, and became very popular again in the 1960s for this reason.

Description The oil is extracted from the dried, fermented leaves of the small shrub and emits an intense, woody, sweet-spicy, balsamic odour. It improves with age and is used as a fixative in perfume.

Therapeutic effects Patchouli is an astringent, and is useful for scalp and skin conditions including dandruff, acne, eczema and scars. It has an uplifting effect for depression and anxiety, and can help alleviate fluid retention.

Uses Inhalation, baths and massage. Small quantities will have a stimulating effect; larger doses sedate. Often worn as a perfume and used for an exotic, sensual massage.

PEPPERMINT
Mentha piperata

Origins The Egyptians used this aromatic herb in flavouring wine and food and valued its menthol content. Culpeper recorded in the seventeenth century that it was the herb most useful for "complaints of the stomach, such as wind and vomiting, for which there are few remedies of greater efficacy".

Description The leaves of peppermint are shorter and broader than spearmint with larger spikes of purple flowers. A British classic, it has spread throughout the world. The almost colourless peppermint oil is distilled from the whole of the partially dried plant and has a strong refreshing fragrance.

Therapeutic effects Excellent for the digestion, as a decongestant, and for skin disorders. Use for colds, flu, flatulence, headaches, indigestion, nausea, toothache and sunburn.

Uses Inhalation, baths and massage. Peppermint oil is still used in gripe water to settle upset stomachs. A few drops on a handkerchief can alleviate headaches and symptoms of sea and travel sickness, as it is refreshing and invigorating. It makes a refreshing skin tonic or bath oil in the summer because of its cooling properties. Used in a footbath it can help sweaty, smelly or tired feet, or in a compress to relieve hot flushes.

Cautionary note For skin complaints do not use in a concentration of more than one per cent as it can cause irritation.

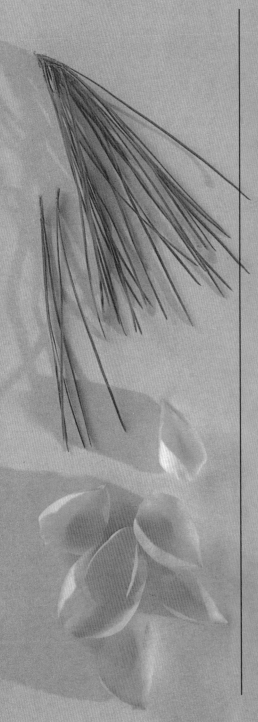

PINE
Pinus sylvestris

Origins The Scandinavians have traditionally used pine in the sauna or steam bath for its refreshing and antiseptic qualities.

Description This species of conifer grows wild all over Europe, North America and the USSR. General pine oil comes from the heart of the wood but the best essences are distilled from the pine needle. The oil has a fresh fragrance with a resinous woody undertone.

Therapeutic effects Acts as an antiseptic, and is particularly valuable for treating the respiratory tract, for bronchitis, catarrh, colds and sinusitis. Will also help relieve cystitis, arthritis and muscular aches and pains.

Uses Inhalation, baths and massage. Widely used to give coniferous fragrance in household products and in some masculine perfumes, this oil is popularly used throughout the cosmetics and pharmaceutical industries in balms, body rubs, soaps and bath oils. The oil can be used as an antiseptic deodorizer (add a few drops to freshen shoes) and in saunas or hot tubs for its invigorating steam.

ROSE
Rosa centifolia, Rosa damascena

Origins The rose has been loved for its fragrance at least since Roman times, when it was used in garlands, scented baths and perfumes, often in ostentatious public displays. But the rose has its private uses too: Cleopatra reputedly carpeted her bedroom in rose petals to aid her seduction of Mark Antony.

Description The Damascena rose is cultivated in Bulgaria. The flowers are picked at dawn and the yellowy-brown oil is extracted within 24 hours. It takes approximately five tons (five tonnes) of blossoms to produce just 2 lb (1 kg) of oil – not surprisingly one of the most expensive in the world. Centifolia roses, also yielding a richly fragrant oil, are cultivated in France, Algeria, Morocco and Eygpt.

Therapeutic effects An aphrodisiac and mood enhancer, rose is a general tonic and fortifier, useful for circulatory problems, constipation, headaches and mental fatigue, menstrual and menopausal problems and skin disorders.

Uses Baths and massage. One of the least toxic of all essences, it is particularly good for older, drier, skins, and is useful for pot pourri or to perfume bed linens and underwear (add a few drops to the final rinse).

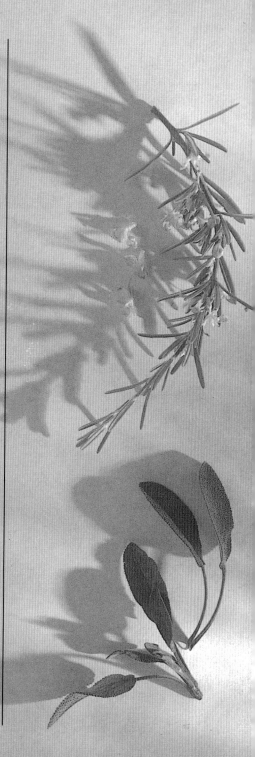

ROSEMARY
Rosmarinus officinalis

Origins First favoured by the Egyptians, rosemary was popular with the Greeks and Romans who believed it symbolized love and death. During the plague it was burned in public places and worn around the neck for its antiseptic qualities.

Description A small shrub, it grows to around three feet (90 cm) high, with grey–green leaves and pale blue–white flowers. The clear oil is steam-distilled from the flowers and leaves, and has a powerful, warm, woody aroma.

Therapeutic effects A good stimulant, especially for the circulation and memory. Also helps alopecia, bronchitis, burns, colds, dandruff, diarrhoea, flatulence, headaches and obesity.

Uses Inhalation, baths and massage. Inhale from a handkerchief to clear headaches and fatigue. In massage it stimulates the lymphatic system.

Cautionary note Use in low concentration, as excessive doses may bring about epileptic fits or convulsions. Do not use in early pregnancy or if you have high blood pressure.

SAGE
Salvia officinalis, Salvia sclarea (Clary sage)

Origins A sacred herb, its properties were used by the Egyptians to help cure infertility in women. The Chinese have used it medicinally for centuries.

Description The many varieties of common sage are all shrub-like herbs with rough, wrinkled leaves. The oil is distilled from the dried leaves and has a powerful, fresh, spicy fragrance with a hint of camphor.

Therapeutic effects A tonic, particularly renowned for regulating menstruation, it can also help relieve arthritis, bacterial infections, throat infections and water retention.

Clary sage (*Salvia sclarea*) is also used for its sedative and euphoric effects, and in treating insomnia, anxiety and depression, as well as menstrual and menopausal problems. It has a spicy fragrance, rather more floral than common sage.

Uses Bathing and massage. A sage bath helps muscular aches and the effects of prolonged stress or mental strain.

Cautionary note In high doses, sage can overstimulate and should be avoided by anyone who suffers from epilepsy. Both sage and clary sage should be avoided in early pregnancy.

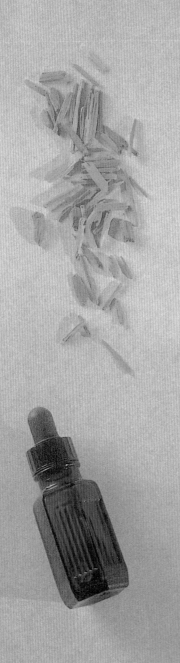

SANDALWOOD
Santalum album

Origins In China, India and Egypt sandalwood was used in perfumes and cosmetics. It has also been prized by furniture makers, and in India many of the temples were built with this lovely wood. Worshippers also covered their bodies with its essence, along with rose, jasmine and narcissus.

Description The evergreen sandalwood tree grows to a height of up to 30 feet (8 metres) in Indonesia, South East Asia and in particular East India. The syrupy, balsamic oil is extracted from the roughly chipped and powdered wood by steam distillation. It has a rich, warm, woody odour. It is used as a fixative in perfumes and gives the lingering classic base notes in many expensive fragrances.

Therapeutic effects Sandalwood's sedative properties are good for treating depression and tension. It is also an expectorant and anti-spasmodic; useful for bronchitis, coughs, nausea, cystitis and skin complaints. Regarded as an aphrodisiac.

Uses Inhalation and massage. Apply in a warm compress to revitalize dehydrated skin. Blends well with neroli and rose. Massage enhances its soothing effects.

TEA TREE
Melaleuca alternifolia

Origins The antiseptic properties of the tea tree were discovered centuries ago by the Aborigines of Australia who used it medicinally for treating sunburn and many bacterial/fungus infections, from ringworm to athlete's foot. It was known as an antidote for venomous snake bites.

Description A native of Australia and Tasmania, it is often referred to as the swamp tree. It produces white hanging flowers on a long spike, but the pale green oil is extracted from the twigs and leaves, which have a strong aromatic odour. The oil itself has a camphorous smell, reminiscent of eucalyptus.

Therapeutic effects A strong disinfectant and antiseptic, it is ideal for skin complaints including athlete's foot, burns, cold sores, mouth ulcers, verrucas, thrush and warts. Also effective for many respiratory complaints.

Uses Inhalation and baths. It can be used to kill fleas on pets but is more commonly used as a deodorizing/antiseptic foot bath. Dab on cold sores. Inhale to alleviate laryngitis and bronchitis. Diluted in water, it can be used as a mouthwash (not swallowed) to soothe ulcers.

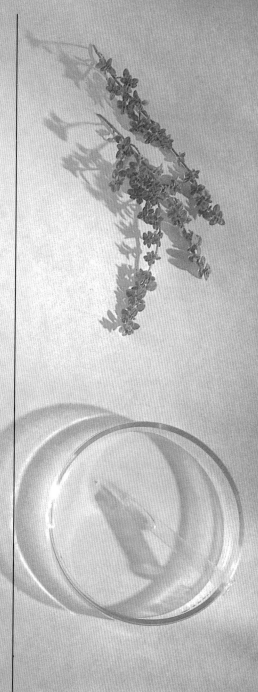

THYME
Thymus vulgaris

Origins The ancient Egyptians incorporated the essential oil of thyme into their embalming fluids. The Greeks drank a herbal infusion of the leaves after banquets to aid digestion. Culpeper considered it a great lung strengthener and a remedy for shortness of breath.

Description This common low-growing wild herb has dark green leaves, woody stalks and small pink flowers. It is cultivated throughout the Mediterranean, Algeria, Yugoslavia and in Egypt for culinary and pharmaceutical uses. The oil is extracted from the whole flowering herb by steam-distillation and has a pungent, sweet herbaceous smell. It is an important component in colognes and herbal perfumes.

Therapeutic effects Helps fatigue and anxiety, but best known as a natural antiseptic for treating coughs and infections of the respiratory tract. Good too for rheumatic aches and for skin problems such as sores and swellings.

Uses Massage and baths. When added to a bath, its invigorating effects help revive tired muscles.

YLANG-YLANG
Cananga odorata

Origins A tropical tree, its first medicinal uses were to treat malaria, soothe insect bites and generally fight infections. Its antiseptic qualities were appreciated but it was also recognized as an aphrodisiac and a tonic to the nervous system. In the past, the flowers were mixed with coconut oil to perfume and condition the body and hair.

Description A native of Indonesia and the Philippines, the ylang-ylang tree reaches a height of 60 feet (10 metres). The yellow flowers are freshly picked in the early morning and the oil extracted by steam-distillation. It has a narcotic, floral-sweet, jasmine-like aroma which adds warmth to perfumes.

Therapeutic effects A great relaxer (if used sparingly) and highly recommended for anxiety, depression, insomnia and frigidity. It also has benefits in treating high blood pressure and skin conditions.

Uses Baths and massage. This oil can soothe away all forms of stress when used as a bath oil or massaged onto the body. Its lasting fragrance is often used in facial and skin preparations, pot pourri and pomanders. It blends well with bergamot, melissa, sandalwood and jasmine.

OILS FOR COMMON PROBLEMS

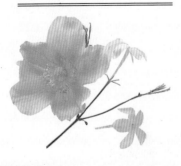

Oil	Type	Acne	Anxiety	Arthritis	Athlete's Foot	Blood pressure: High	Low	Body odour	Bronchitis	Cellulite	Colds/chills
Basil	R, U		✿						✿		✿
Bay	R			✿					✿	✿	
Benzoin	S			✿					✿	✿	✿
Bergamot	R, U	✿	✿								
Cedarwood	R	✿							✿		
Chamomile	R	✿	✿	✿							
Cinnamon	R							✿			✿
Comfrey	R				✿						
Cypress	R		✿					✿		✿	
Eucalyptus	S	✿		✿					✿		✿
Fennel	S										
Frankincense	R										✿
Geranium	R, U		✿								✿
Hyssop	R, S						✿	✿	✿		
Jasmine	R		✿								
Juniper	R, U	✿	✿							✿	
Lavender	R, U	✿	✿	✿	✿	✿			✿	✿	
Lemon	S	✿						✿			
Lemongrass	S	✿			✿			✿			
Marjoram	R			✿	✿	✿				✿	
Melissa	R, U		✿			✿					
Myrrh	S								✿	✿	✿
Neroli	R		✿					✿			
Orange	U		✿			✿					
Parsley	S										
Patchouli	R	✿	✿			✿				✿	
Peppermint	S							✿	✿	✿	
Pine	S			✿					✿	✿	✿
Rose	R		✿	✿							
Rosemary	S							✿		✿	✿
Sage	S			✿	✿			✿		✿	
Clary Sage	R, S		✿			✿					
Sandalwood	R	✿	✿							✿	
Tea Tree	S				✿					✿	✿
Thyme	S		✿							✿	
Ylang-Ylang	R		✿			✿					

	Cystitis	Dandruff	Depression	Diarrhoea	Eczema	Fainting	Flatulence	Haemorrhoids	Hayfever	Headache	Hormonal regulation	Indigestion	Influenza	Insomnia	Menopausal problems	Menstrual problems (general)	Irregular periods	Painful periods	Mental fatigue	Muscular aches	Nausea	Obesity	Pre-menstrual syndrome	Rheumatism	Sexual problems	Sinusitus	Stress	Throat infections	Travel sickness	Varicose veins	Warts	Water retention
			❀			❀				❀		❀	❀			❀				❀		❀		❀								
																								❀								
	❀																															
	❀		❀				❀																					❀				
		❀			❀								❀											❀								
❀			❀	❀	❀				❀	❀	❀	❀	❀		❀	❀	❀	❀	❀				❀	❀			❀					
			❀									❀						❀				❀									
			❀										❀			❀		❀													
	❀		❀	❀	❀			❀					❀	❀	❀		❀		❀	❀	❀	❀		❀	❀	❀			❀		❀
	❀			❀				❀	❀	❀		❀				❀		❀				❀		❀		❀		❀			
❀						❀							❀							❀	❀										
													❀													❀					
	❀	❀	❀	❀						❀					❀							❀		❀		❀	❀				❀
						❀			❀				❀	❀		❀															
		❀		❀																		❀		❀							
	❀	❀		❀	❀		❀						❀			❀	❀	❀				❀	❀				❀			❀	❀
	❀	❀	❀	❀		❀		❀			❀		❀		❀	❀	❀			❀	❀			❀		❀	❀	❀	❀	❀	❀
	❀		❀																			❀				❀	❀	❀			
			❀									❀		❀											❀	❀	❀			
❀			❀					❀		❀		❀		❀			❀			❀				❀		❀					
			❀						❀	❀	❀	❀		❀	❀	❀	❀	❀						❀			❀				
			❀	❀		❀			❀			❀												❀							
		❀				❀							❀	❀								❀	❀		❀						
❀		❀				❀					❀	❀											❀								
	❀																														❀
	❀	❀		❀																	❀			❀							
		❀			❀	❀	❀	❀		❀		❀									❀				❀			❀	❀		
❀									❀									❀	❀			❀		❀							❀
❀		❀						❀				❀			❀	❀	❀		❀		❀		❀			❀	❀				
❀		❀	❀		❀	❀				❀			❀		❀	❀	❀		❀	❀	❀	❀	❀			❀			❀		❀
	❀		❀									❀		❀	❀	❀			❀					❀							❀
			❀				❀					❀		❀	❀	❀															
	❀	❀	❀		❀			❀					❀									❀		❀	❀	❀					
		❀												❀										❀		❀		❀			
						❀										❀			❀				❀	❀	❀						
		❀																				❀									

THE ESSENTIAL MASSAGE

An aromatherapy massage using essential oils is a therapeutic treatment for both mind and body which works mainly on the nervous system. Aromatherapy is both holistic and practical in that it helps to protect the body's life-saving immune system and energize or stabilize emotions. It is often called the "sensual science" because it combines the powers of touch with the sense of smell. More effectively than any other massage, aromatherapy can either relax or stimulate the body and mind. The highly potent essential oils penetrate the body via the skin and are also inhaled as the massage progresses.

SETTING UP

Any massage is relaxing but you can enhance the experience by following a few simple steps to help create the right mood.

An aromatherapist uses a massage bench, but at home you can work comfortably on a cushioned floor or a futon (Japanese mattress). An ordinary bed is not really firm enough. Prepare the floor or surface with a large cotton sheet covered with a bath towel. You should also have to hand a pillow, a large wrap-around towel for the body, and a warm blanket or even a hot-water bottle by the feet.

RELAXING YOUR PARTNER

Additional touches help to establish a calming atmosphere. You could fragrance the room with a burner, using a relaxing oil, and switch on some background music: play instrumental tracks, as voices can distract any train of thought.

The room temperature should be warm. Once the oils are gently massaged in, the whole body responds by slowing down and, although the skin may feel warm to touch, the body feels colder. It is important to keep your partner comfortable, so offer to cover parts that are not being worked on if you think your partner may be getting cold. Being at ease with one another is an important part of any treatment.

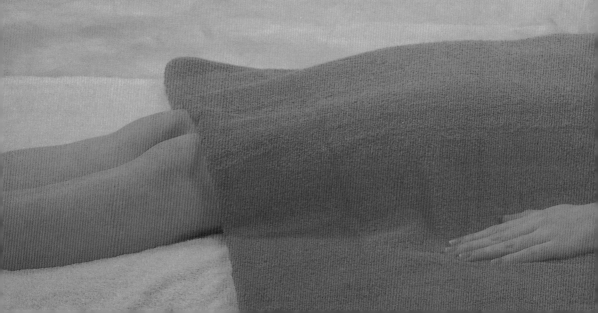

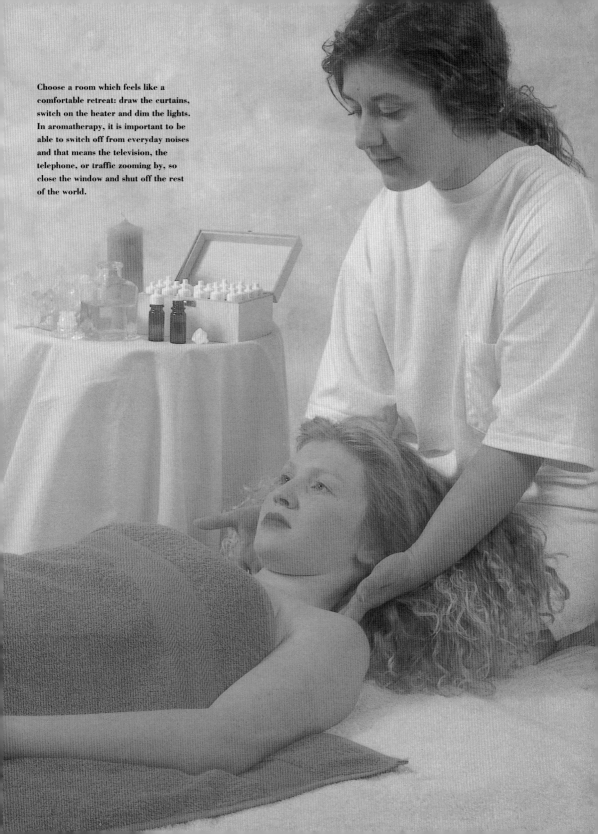

Choose a room which feels like a
comfortable retreat: draw the curtains,
switch on the heater and dim the lights.
In aromatherapy, it is important to be
able to switch off from everyday noises
and that means the television, the
telephone, or traffic zooming by, so
close the window and shut off the rest
of the world.

ABOUT THE TREATMENT

A complete aromatherapy massage takes just under an hour from top to toe. It is important to find out before massage about physical aches and pains, in particular back injuries, recent operations or whether the person you are massaging is in an "emotional" state of mind at the time.

GIVING THE MASSAGE

● Make sure you have read through the step-by-step instructions several times to familiarize yourself with the sequence. You don't want to keep stopping to refer to the book.
● Try out the movements on parts of your own body to get a sense of how the strokes should feel and how much pressure to use.
● Massage movements should be slow and gentle to help relaxation and eliminate tension which tightens the muscles.
● Remember that the movements should flow into each other. If you find you have missed out a step or gone on to the wrong part of the body, don't panic. Finish the part you are working on before going back to it, or leave it out altogether, rather than interrupting the flow of the massage.
● When you give the massage, make sure *you* are relaxed and comfortable, as well as the person you're working on, or you will transmit your own tensions to your partner and it will not be an effective massage.
● Try to maintain contact with your partner's body as much as possible; even as you move into a different position try to keep a hand on the body.
● When massaging different parts of the body keep the areas not being worked on covered with a large towel or blanket. The heat helps the body to absorb the oils.

CHOOSING THE ESSENTIAL OIL

 romatherapists never start a massage immediately. In order to provide the most effective treatment, the therapist has to ascertain the state of mind and body of the individual, and establish whether there are any specific problems to attend to. Is the problem physical? Is it mental? Is it a combination of both? To help them to treat a wide variety of complaints, aromatherapists have many oils at their fingertips, but they never mix or use them until they have worked out a prescription for the receiver's individual needs.

Mixing the oils is a trained art, yet there are simple recipes you can use at home to deal with specific problems from muscular aches and pains to headaches and stress. With potent essential oils it is far better to use less, rather than more, so if in doubt, start the massage technique with a base oil like sweet almond and add two or three drops of just one essential oil. Lavender, rosemary and geranium are good all-purpose oils, or use chamomile for particularly sensitive skin.

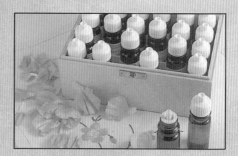

APPLYING THE OILS

eep the oil in an easy dispenser or bowl so you don't have to worry about lids during the massage. But keep the oil covered in some way as essential oils will quickly evaporate.

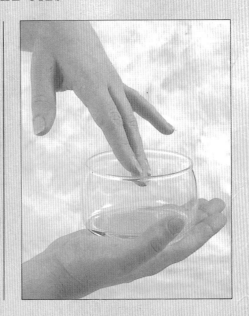

● Always warm your hands before applying oils.

● Some therapists recommend warming the oil in your hands before applying it to the body as a courtesy to the recipient. Others advise against this on the grounds that it hastens evaporation of the essential oil and that the oil takes on your own energy rather than your partner's.

● If the part of the body you're working on is particularly hairy or the skin is very dry you will need to apply more oil.

● Keep your touch light and sensitive. Remember that your hands are the main channel of communication.

● If the recipient's back is stressed in any way, place a pillow under the knees when lying on the back, and under the pelvis when lying on the stomach.

● Wear loose comfortable clothing to give the massage, so your movements are not hampered.

● If oil is accidentally spilt on clothing, dab off quickly with a tissue. It will soon evaporate, but it may leave a stain so rinse out clothing in warm soapy water.

● For complete relaxation avoid chatting during the massage: play music if you don't like silence. But do encourage feedback from your partner – you must be told if something doesn't feel good.

● Ensure that the person you are going to work on is given the following set of guidelines.

RECEIVING THE MASSAGE

Before the Massage
● Have a cool shower or wash before a massage. Do not soak in a hot bath, or the oils will immediately seep into the skin.

● Don't use an underarm deodorant or body spray during the treatment, as this will block the effect of the oils.

● Don't have a large meal just before an aromatherapy massage as the body's systems will have to work too hard at digesting to be thoroughly relaxed.

● Don't drink alcohol before a treatment.

● Don't have a massage if you have flu or a fever or any serious condition (see Cautions). Wait until you are over the worst and then let an aromatherapy treatment help restore your system's balance.

After the Massage
● Drink a glass of still water immediately after a treatment.

● Lie still for at least five minutes before getting up.

● Don't bathe or shower for at least twelve hours after a treatment to allow the oils to be absorbed by the skin and begin the all-important work of detoxifying the body.

● Drink plenty of water for the rest of the day as the kidneys will be active in eliminating the toxins.

● Avoid alcohol for at least 12 hours after the treatment to give the body a chance to detoxify thoroughly.

THE MASSAGE STEP-BY-STEP

Following your assessment, select the oils you are going to use and blend 10–15 drops of your chosen oils with four tablespoons of base oil.

The massage starts with your partner lying face down, with the back uncovered and the rest of the body covered with a towel or light blanket.

ESTABLISHING CONTACT

Take a few moments to create a bond of communication with your partner and to prepare yourself for the massage. Focus or "centre" yourself by becoming aware of your whole body and its role in giving the massage, and letting go of outside concerns to concentrate on the task in hand.

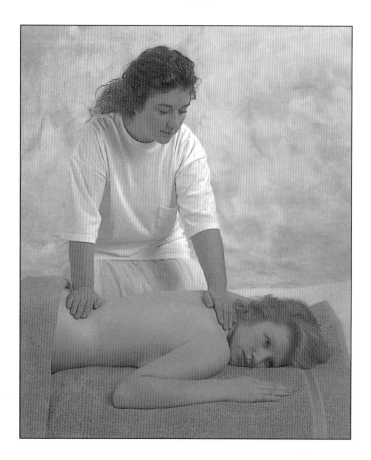

CAUTIONS

Aromatherapy is an holistic therapy in that it works on the person as a whole. Though it is an excellent way of treating minor ailments, stress and negative emotional states, it is not a substitute for conventional medical treatment. If symptoms persist, always consult a medical doctor.

Never attempt to treat the following conditions:
● cancer
● progressive neural disorders
● heart conditions
● advanced asthmatic conditions
● post-operative states
● severe varicose veins
● very high blood pressure
● epilepsy

For oils to avoid during pregnancy *see* Pregnancy Treatments.

Left: With your partner face down, rest one hand lightly at the base of the neck (the occipital bone) and place your other hand on the lower back (the sacral area). Hold the position for a count of 20, while you focus on your breathing and clear your mind. This is carried out with dry hands.

THE LEG

EFFLEURAGE (SMOOTHING STROKE)

This is a smooth, sliding movement which soothes the skin and distributes the oil. Always worked in the direction of the heart, effleurage improves circulation, lymph flow and the function of the muscles. It is used between movements throughout the massage to provide continuity and to prepare a new area with oil.

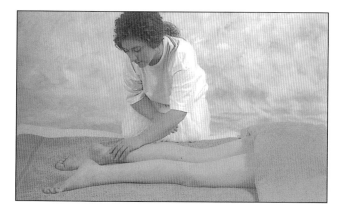

1 *Seated to the side of your partner, begin with one hand at the heel, brushing in an upward, sweeping movement to the buttock ridge and sliding round to the thigh.*

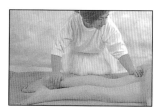

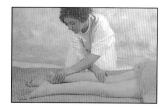

2 *As the first hand comes round the thigh, place the other hand at the heel and brush with an upward sweep, ending at the back of the knee.*

3 *As the second hand comes off, cross the first hand over and begin the movement again from the heel up to the thigh.*

Repeat the sequence about six or seven times, keeping the movements continuous and flowing, and then repeat on the other leg.

ANKLE THUMBING

The ankles are an important centre of energy, and this movement helps to relieve congestion.

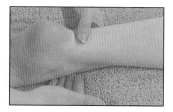

1 *Sitting at your partner's feet, cradle one ankle gently with your hands, allowing the thumbs to sit naturally above the heel.*

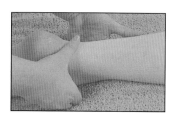

2 *Keeping the rest of the hand still, apply a light pressure with the thumb as it brushes in an upward and outward movement.*

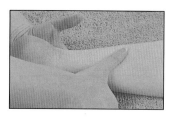

3 *Repeat with alternate thumbs, continuing in a rhythmic sequence for about 30 seconds.*

FLUSHING

Flushing drains the lymph channels and stimulates the circulation.
This movement should not be used on anyone with severe varicose veins.

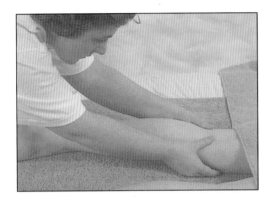 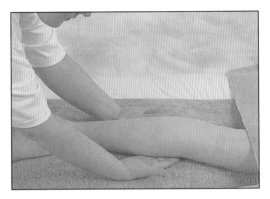

1 *Sitting at your partner's feet,*
gently slide the thumbs up the
middle of the leg, ending at the back
of the knee.

2 *Slowly bring the hands back*
down to the ankles by brushing
down the sides of the calf muscle,
taking care not to drag.

Repeat the movement five or six times.

KNEADING

Move back round to the side of the leg for this movement. It is particularly
effective for relieving tension at the back of the legs.

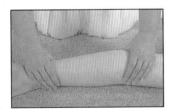 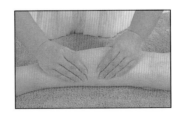 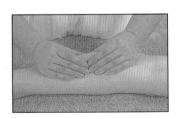

1 *Place the hands gently on the*
calf, one at the top and one
just above the ankle.

2 *Grasp the calf muscle firmly*
with both hands and slide
them toward the centre of the calf,
lifting the muscle.

3 *Using gentle pressure, knead*
the area by bringing the
fingers and thumbs together and
raising the muscle further.

Continue kneading for about 30 seconds.

WRINGING

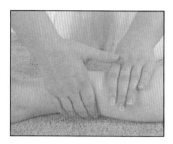
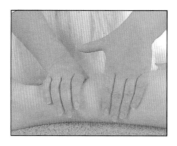
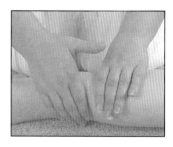

1 *Place the hands on opposite sides of the calf, just above the ankle. Gently glide the hands past each other so the heel of one hand is pushing away from you while the other hand is pulling.*

2 *Keep the thumb of the pulling hand raised so the thumbs don't collide as they pass each other each time.*

3 *The hands alternate the pushing and pulling as you work all the way up the calf and down again. The pressure should be firm but gentle.*

Clear these movements by flushing through again from ankle to back of knee.

THUMBING THE KNEE

This is the same action as the thumbing performed at the ankle base. It is helpful for people who suffer from cold feet as it stimulates the circulation.

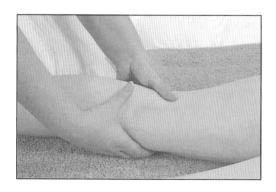
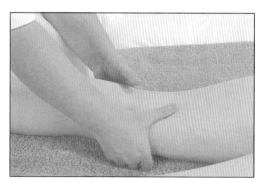

1 *Cup the hands gently around the knee, allowing the thumbs to sit naturally on the fleshy part at the back of the knee.*

2 *With the same thumbing movement used on the ankles, brush one thumb upward and outward, covering the full width of the knee, and follow immediately with the opposite thumb.*

43

FLUSHING

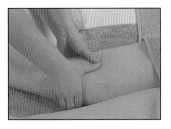

*Flush through with the thumbs
together from the back of the knee
to the top of the thigh.*

WRINGING

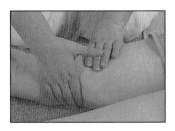

*Wring the leg from the knee to the
top of the thigh with the same
action as used on the lower leg.*

THIGH PUSH

*This knuckling movement is very effective for breaking down cellulite,
helping to disperse the fatty tissue and improve the circulation.*

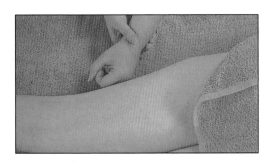

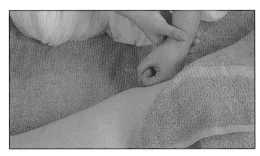

1 *With the supporting hand
wrapped around the wrist of
the working hand for stability,
place the clenched fist on the side
of the thigh, just above the knee.*

2 *Drag the fist slowly up the
side of the thigh toward the
hip bone. This is not a heavy action
– all you need is gentle pressure.*

Repeat five or six times, working slightly different parts of the thigh each time.

Finish the leg massage by repeating the opening effluerage *movement
and then repeat all the steps on the other leg.*

*Cover the legs with towels before proceeding to the
next stage. An extra blanket or hot water bottle
at the feet might also be appreciated.*

BACK MASSAGE

*The back carries a lot of strain and these relaxing movements are often
the most appreciated part of the massage. Don't be tempted to use too
much pressure: it is better to keep the strokes broad and flowing.*

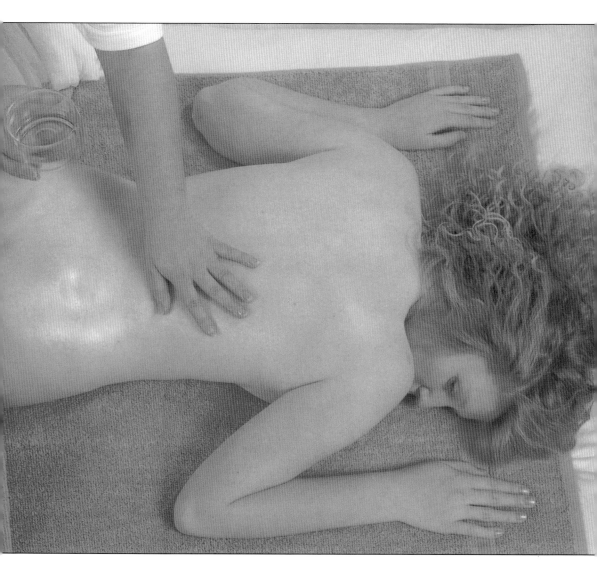

*Seated to the side of your partner, apply oil evenly over
the back with smooth upward strokes, following the
direction of the lymph flow.*

45

FIGURE-OF-EIGHT

This sequence loosens the tissue all over the back and helps to stimulate
blood and lymph flow, and relieve tension.

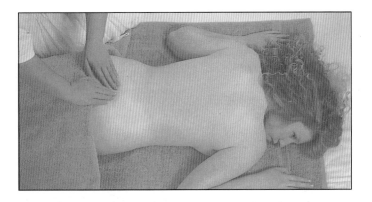

You should be kneeling level with
the buttocks, facing the head so
that you can lean into the
movement and reach the shoulders
without straining.

1 To begin this large sweeping
movement, place both hands on
the lower back, just above the base
of the spine, fingers pointing
toward the head.

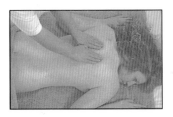

2 Slide both hands all the way
up the sides of the spine to just
below the base of the neck.

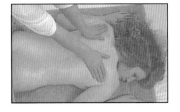

3 Move the hands out around
the shoulders and in toward
each other across the upper back.

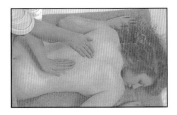

4 As the hands pass each other,
cross the right arm over the left
and continue gliding.

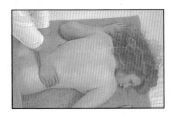

5 With arms still crossed, reach
down around the waist.

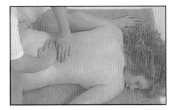

6 Pull the flesh up firmly
around the waist and then
gradually release the sides as the
palms glide to the middle of the
lower back and pass each other.

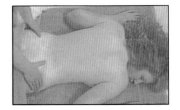

7 Continue the movement by
sliding the palms out around
the hips and complete the figure-of-
eight by returning the hands to the
starting position.

Repeat six times, always keeping the movements broad and flowing.

FANNING

This action works on the nerves along the spine and helps to disperse the fluid that accumulates in the back tissue as a result of tension. The effect is wonderfully relaxing.

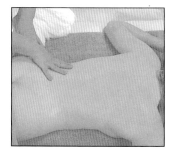

1 Place one hand on the lower back, at the base of the spine. The fingers should be splayed open, with the index finger pointing to the side of the spine.

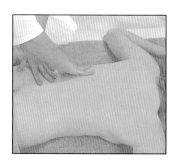

2 Fan the hand round in an upward and outward motion away from the spine. The other hand follows on the same side as the first completes the movement. Work all the way up the side of the spine, alternating hands.

Repeat the steps four or five times before moving round to work on the other side of the spine.

BUTTERFLY SHOULDERS

Before being given an aromatherapy massage, always wash off any anti-perspirant or deodorant. This is particularly important for this movement as it drains the lymph towards the major lymph glands in the armpits – the axillary glands. This movement relaxes the shoulder and disperses tension.

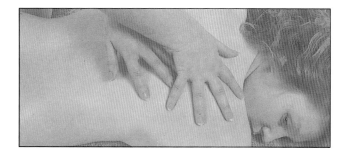

1 Place one hand at the bottom of the shoulder blade (scapula) with fingers splayed and the second hand poised to follow on the same side.

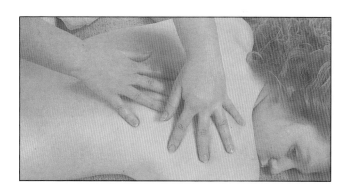

2 Brush the hand up and out in a smooth fanning movement. Follow with the second hand, work all round the shoulder blade and out over the shoulder, toward the armpit.

Repeat the whole movement four times, then work on the other shoulder.

FOREARM SWEEP

Kneeling at the side of your partner, turn the head away from you.

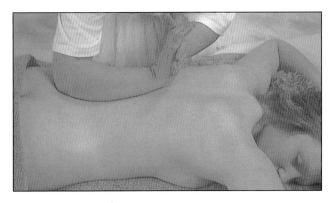

1 *Place your forearm alongside the spine with your elbow just above the buttocks. Clasp the working hand with your other hand for support and stability.*

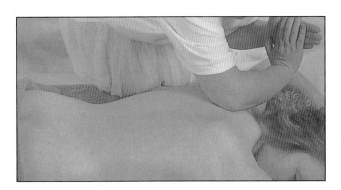

2 *Using the flat bone of the forearm (the ulna), slide all the way up the side of the spine to the top of the shoulder ridge.*

Lift the arm off gently and repeat twice from the beginning.

Then turn your partner's head and work on the other side of the spine, using the opposite forearm.

DRAINING

Sit to the side of your partner, facing across the back.

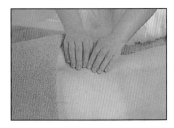

1 *With hands together and palms raised, place the fingertips at the side of the spine, just above the coccyx (tail bone).*

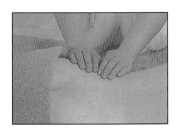

2 *Keeping the fingers together, pull them toward you down the side of the back.*

Repeat the movement all the way up the spine, ending at the base of the neck so the final movement pulls across the shoulders toward the glands in the armpit.

Repeat with the other side of the spine. You can work the opposite side without changing your position by reaching across and brushing away from the spine, or you can move around your partner and repeat as above, if it feels more comfortable.

KNEADING THE NECK

This gentle petrissage *movement releases tension and helps disperse the fatty deposits that can build up in this sensitive area.*

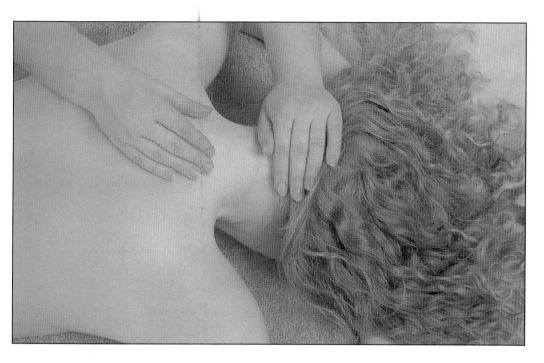

Your partner should rest facing down with forehead on hands, so that you can work your fingers into the base of the neck. Smooth the hair away from the neck.

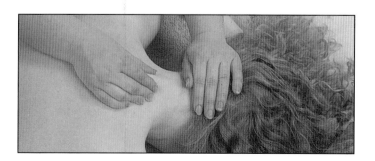

Resting one hand gently on the back of the head, use the other hand to pull up and knead the muscles in the base of the neck (the occipitals), rolling the muscle between the thumb and the other fingers.

FRONTAL MASSAGE

Help your partner to turn over onto their back, and ensure he or she is comfortable.
Provide cushions or rolled towels for any parts that need support,
such as behind the legs or neck. Cover the body up to the neck
with a towel or blanket to keep your partner warm.

SPINAL STRETCH

This movement is not suitable for people suffering from severe
back problems, though it helps relieve minor aches and stiffness.

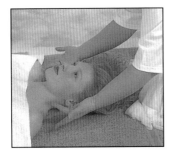

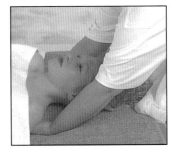

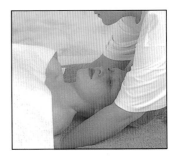

1 *Seated at your partner's head, place the hands to the sides of the neck, palms up, with the middle fingers lifted, to prepare for the movement.*

2 *Slide the hands underneath the back, just between the shoulder blades so the middle fingers are pressing on either side of the spine.*

3 *Gently lift the torso so the rib cage rises, maintaining the pressure from the middle fingers.*

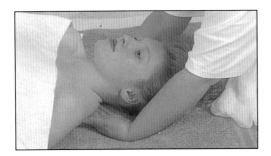

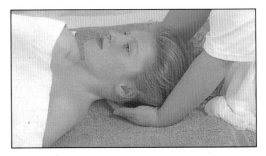

4 *Slowly pull your fingers up the sides of the spine. When you reach the top of the neck, hold for a count of two and then release. Repeat three times in all.*

5 *Finish the movement by cradling the head gently with both hands.*

THE FACE

This treatment is a great boost to the circulation, and the complexion will improve with each treatment.

Seated at the head, prepare the face for the massage with a simple refreshing cleanser, using upward and outward strokes. Apply a small amount of facial oil to the face and neck with flowing movements.

TAKE CARE

Even when diluted, essential oils are extremely potent so work carefully around the eye area. If the oil accidentally makes contact with the eye, apply a few drops of pure sweet almond oil to dissipate it. Never wash the eyes with water.

FOREHEAD STROKE

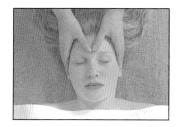

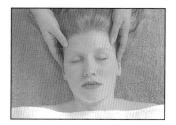

1 *Rest your thumbs on the centre of the forehead, just above the eyebrows, with the palms supporting the sides of the head. The stroke should be kept light and sensitive as the facial skin is very delicate.*

2 *Slowly draw the thumbs out toward the temples and down to the sides of the ears. Repeat the stroke several times, moving the starting position up a little each time until you reach the hairline.*

DRAINING THE CHEEKS

This sequence of raking movements stimulates the lymphatic flow in the face, improving the complexion, clearing the sinuses and releasing tension.

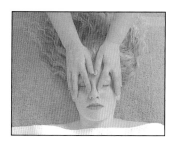

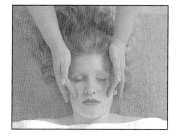

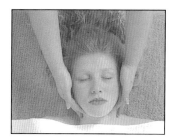

1 *Place the index fingers on either side of the nostrils and hold for a count of five.*

2 *Slide the fingers out and down to the ears. Lift the fingers and replace by the nostril. Sweep in a slightly narrower curve to reach the jawbone just below the ears.*

3 *Repeat with successively smaller curves, ending by tracing the laughter lines around the mouth, downward to the sides of the chin.*

CHIN MASSAGE

This not only tones the jawline, but also stimulates the energy points that govern the stomach and small intestine.

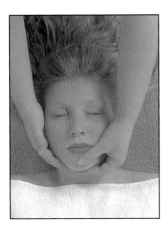

1 *Place the thumbs on the chin, allowing the rest of the fingers to cradle the jaw.*

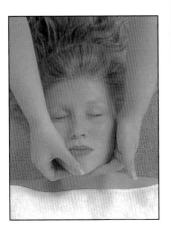

2 *Brush alternate thumbs down and outward, with a light stroke. Repeat the movement six or seven times with each thumb.*

NECK SWEEP

This is an extremely soothing stroke which improves the tone of the muscles as well as flushing the neck.

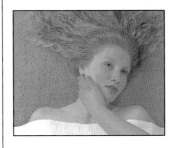

1,2 *Above and right: Apply a little facial oil to the neck, upper chest and shoulder areas using the flat of the hand. Gently brush down with the hand from the side of the ear out to the shoulder, using a broad sweeping stroke to cover the area.*

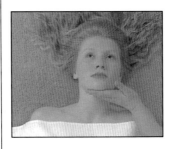

3 *Repeat the movement working round the front of the neck, down from the chin to the top of the chest, and then sweep from the other ear to the shoulder.*

The sequence of sweeps round the whole neck should be repeated three times.

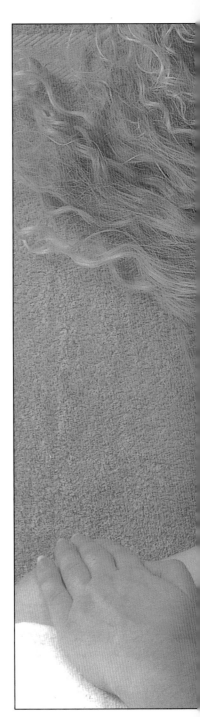

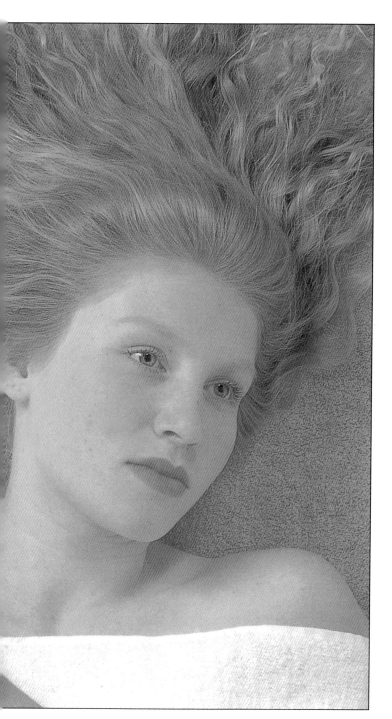

FANNING THE SHOULDERS

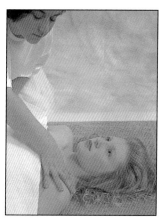

1 *With fingers spread, brush with the flat of the hand across from the breastbone and out over the shoulders.*

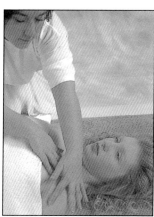

2 *The second hand follows closely behind the first, so they are draining simultaneously toward the armpit.*

Repeat twice before moving onto the other shoulder.

STOMACH AREA

ABDOMEN

1 *Left: Apply a little oil evenly over the stomach. Place the palm of a hand on the centre of the abdomen.*

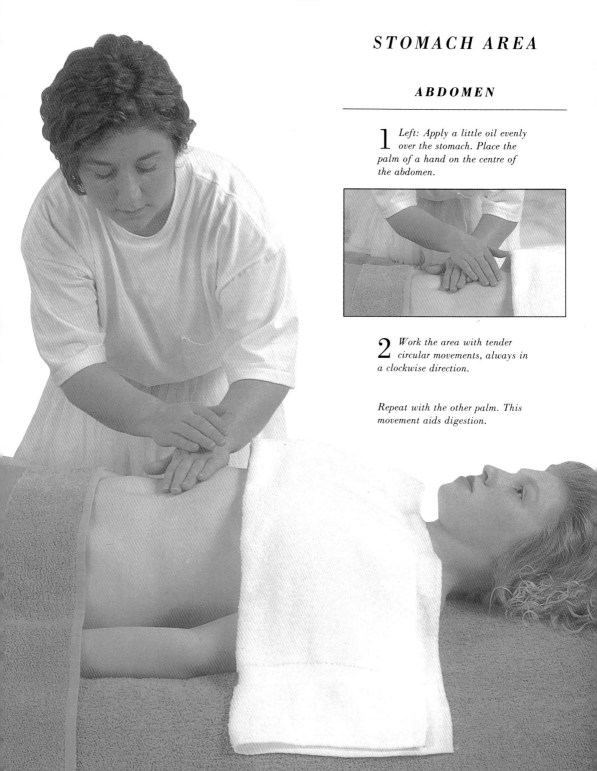

2 *Work the area with tender circular movements, always in a clockwise direction.*

Repeat with the other palm. This movement aids digestion.

RIB-CAGE SWEEP

This movement helps to cleanse the stomach and spleen by pushing the lymph away from these areas.

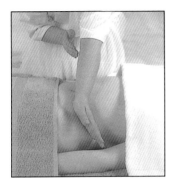

1 *Starting with the outer edge of the hand placed at the centre of the rib-cage, sweep away from you, following the line of the ribs with a long sweeping movement out to the waist.*

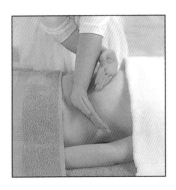

2 *As the first hand finishes the movement, the other hand follows on the same side.*

Repeat the movement with both hands six or seven times and then move around the body to work the other side of the rib-cage.

WAIST PULLS

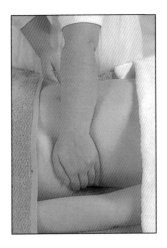 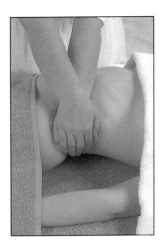

1 *Reach across your partner, placing a firm grip round the waist with one hand. Reinforce your grip by placing your other hand on top of the first hand.*

2 *Lift the waist by pulling your partner's body-weight toward you, then gently release while sliding the hands around the hipbone. This cleanses the liver and gall bladder.*

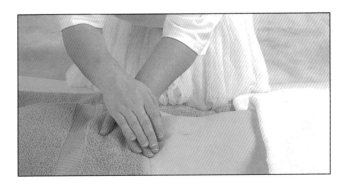

3 *Complete the movement by sliding the hands across and around the pelvis, draining toward the major glands in the groin. Be careful not to dig with the fingers as this is an*

extremely tender area. Keep the pressure light and even over the whole hand. This is particularly beneficial for women who suffer from menstrual problems.

Repeat five or six times before moving round to the other side of the body.

FRONT OF LEGS

EFFLEURAGE

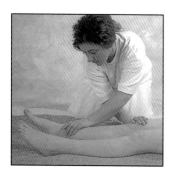

Apply oil to both legs using an effleurage *movement working up from the ankles, as used on the back of the legs.*

Repeat the effleurage *strokes sequence several times to ensure an even distribution of oil.*

LEG STRETCH

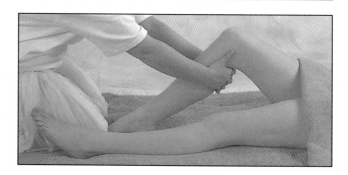

Supporting the leg at the ankle and behind the knee, bend the leg up and place it in line with the shoulder.
 Clasp the hands around the back of the knee. Ask your partner to inhale deeply, then pull the calf muscle toward you.

Hold for a slow count of three. As your partner breathes out, release the pull on the calf.

Repeat the whole movement three times, then gently lay the leg down and repeat the stretch on the other leg.

ARMS AND HANDS

EFFLEURAGE

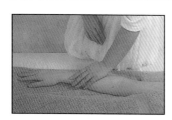

1 Seated to the side of your partner, move the arm slightly away from the body. Apply the oil by sweeping from just above the wrist, up to the shoulder and round.

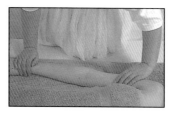

2 As the first hand comes off the arm, the other hand starts at the wrist and sweeps upward to the gland sited in the elbow joint.

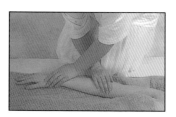

3 The first arm crosses the second as it reaches the elbow and again sweeps from wrist to shoulder.

Repeat six or seven times.

You can follow the effleurage *with flushing to the inside
of the arm, using the same movements performed on the leg, working
from the wrist to the elbow.
Before going on to the second arm, massage the hand of the first arm.*

HAND MASSAGE

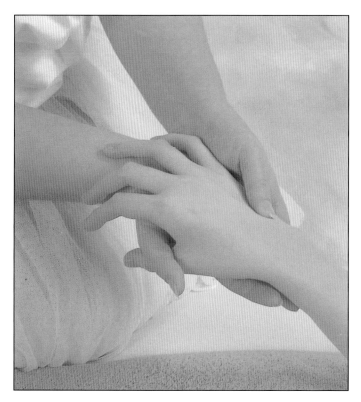

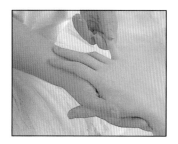

2 *Pull back to the fingers, gently
massaging the joints between
your thumb and forefinger as you
draw towards the tips. Finish with
a slight pull to the finger to stretch
it out.*

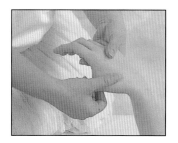

1 *Resting your partner's hand
palm down over your own
palm, use small brushing*

*movements with your thumbs to
work upward between the joints of
the fingers toward the wrist.*

3 *Repeat with each finger,
finishing with the thumb.*

Now repeat the movements on the other arm and hand.

*To finish the massage, cover your partner to the neck, check he or she
is warm and comfortable, and leave to rest for a minimum of five minutes (up to
15 minutes is preferable). Upon returning, help your partner to sit up
carefully and offer a glass of water.*

PREGNANCY TREATMENTS

Pregnancy can be one of the most exciting and fulfilling times of a woman's life. The joy of bringing another human being into the world creates a tremendous feeling of contentment and anticipation, but it is also a time of great physical and emotional upheaval. Together with the ever-important trio of exercise, good diet and rest, essential oils can play an important role in helping a woman cope with the stresses of nine months of pregnancy, the pain of labour and post-natal recovery.

COMMON AILMENTS

Surging hormone levels and changes in your swelling body can bring a host of discomforts, many of which can be alleviated by aromatherapy treatments and other simple steps.

Backache
The lower back region takes a lot of strain during pregnancy, and will benefit from a firm massage with four drops each of lavender and sandalwood in two tablespoons of base oil. Six drops of lavender in the bath will help to soothe away the aches.

Morning Sickness
Eat little and often during the day, avoiding junk food and heavy meals late at night. Choose fresh foods which are free from preservatives or chemicals. Try herbal tea infusions such as chamomile, peppermint or orange blossom, which are good for the digestion.

Heartburn
Avoid heavy meals and particularly rich, spicy foods. Peppermint tea infusions help, and you can rub the solar plexus with a blend of two drops each of lemon and peppermint essential oils in one tablespoon of base oil.

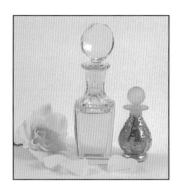

Spoil yourself with the luxurious and relaxing scent of rose for body and facial oils, to keep your spirits up during pregnancy.

Sore Breasts
These need extra care and attention during pregnancy as they expand. Use a gentle massage oil with rose and orange, three drops of each in one tablespoon of sweet almond oil; or if breasts are swollen, make a cool compress using rosewater and place over the breasts while having an afternoon rest. Sweet almond oil on its own is excellent for sore, cracked nipples during breast-feeding. Never use pure essential oils on the breasts during this period as they can easily be transferred to the baby while feeding.

Constipation
Make sure your diet contains plenty of fresh and high fibre foods and drink plenty of still water. Tension can also be a contributory factor, so try a relaxing bath with three drops of lavender and four drops of rose. Massage your abdomen and the small of the back with a blend of four drops of chamomile or orange in one tablespoon of base oil.

Sleep Problems
In the last few months of pregnancy, with the baby kicking and other discomforts, it is often difficult to get a good night's sleep. A relaxing bath with neroli and rose is soothing, and you can add ylang-ylang for its calming, sedative effect – a maximum of eight drops in total. Two drops of rose or lavender on the edge of the pillowcase will help induce sleep.

Stretch Marks
When the stretched skin returns to the body's normal shape it can leave tiny jagged scars. A daily massage around the hips and expanding tummy, using five drops of lavender in one tablespoon of jojoba, wheatgerm or evening primrose oil, will help keep skin smooth and supple. Start around the fifth month of

pregnancy and continue after the birth until you return to your normal weight.

Swollen Ankles

These can be reduced with a cool to warm footbath of benzoin, rose and orange. Add two drops of each directly to the bowl or mix with one tablespoon of base carrier oil such as sesame seed. Rest with feet raised on cushions or pillows.

Varicose Veins

During pregnancy the blood flow to the legs is often slowed down, causing the veins to dilate. Two drops each of cypress, lemongrass and lavender, mixed with two tablespoons of apricot kernel base oil, can be smoothed gently over the legs for relief. If veins are prominent then one of the best oils for the circulation is geranium, though this should always be very dilute for use in pregnancy. Add four drops to the bath or to one tablespoon of carrier oil to massage the leg with upward movements. Do not work directly on the veins or apply too much pressure to the leg.

LABOUR

To create a relaxing atmosphere in the labour room, use a few drops of lavender in a fragrancer, or try rose, neroli or ylang-ylang to fortify you as the labour pro-gresses. Any of these oils can be used in a massage blend for the lower back to help with con-tractions. If labour is progressing slowly, try marjoram as a massage oil or compress across the abdomen to stimulate contractions.

AFTER THE BIRTH

The "baby blues" often occur around the third or fourth day after childbirth, though some

CAUTIONS

The following oils should be avoided during pregnancy (particularly the first five months) because of their strong diuretic properties or tendency to induce menstruation:

Bay · Basil · Clary Sage · Comfrey Fennel · Hyssop · Juniper Marjoram · Melissa · Myrrh Rosemary · Thyme · Sage

Use all essential oils in half the usual quantity during pregnancy and take extra care in handling them. Ensure that the oils you are using are pure essential oils, as adulterated blends

or synthetic oils can sometimes have less predictable effects.

If you have a history of miscarriage you could also avoid chamomile and lavender for the first few months, although in general these are excellent oils for pregnancy.

Because of their potentially toxic nature and strong abortive qualities the following oils should *never* be used except by a qualified aromatherapist, and must be avoided during pregnancy:

Oreganum · Pennyroyal · St John's Wort · Tansy · Wormwood

women can suffer a more severe form of post-natal depression for up to a year. A bath of jasmine and ylang-ylang will help you feel better, or use a body oil of chamomile, geranium and orange (5 drops to two tablespoons of sweet almond oil), which is a good mix for hormonal imbalance.

To ease any perineal pains, a bath with lavender is soothing. Tea tree can also be added, since this is a powerful antiseptic and helps heal internal wounds and stitches.

Recommended Oils for Pregnancy
Chamomile · Geranium (in low doses) *· Lavender · Lemon · Neroli Orange · Rose · Sandalwood*

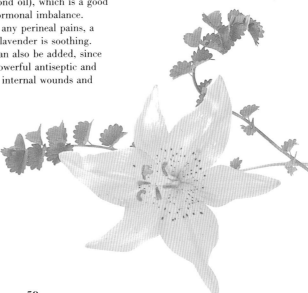

PREGNANCY MASSAGE

These simple touch massage movements can help to relieve many of the stresses and discomforts of pregnancy, and the back massage is particularly welcome during labour. The basic essential oil massage is modified in various ways to take account of the pregnant condition.

● Check the box on the previous page to find which oils are suitable and which are to be avoided.
● Use a lower concentration of essential oil to base oil; $\frac{1}{2}$–1 per cent is ideal.
● Keep strokes lighter than usual.
● In addition to the steps suggested, you can incorporate a facial and gentle breast massage.
● It is particularly important to observe the rest period after the massage and to help your partner get up gently.
● The positions you work in need to be adapted for a pregnant woman, as she cannot lie out straight on her front or back and needs to be well supported.

THE BACK

After about the fourth month of pregnancy it becomes uncomfortable to lie on the stomach, so work with your partner sitting up with a towel-wrapped pillow or back of a chair to lean over for support.

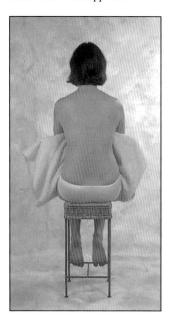

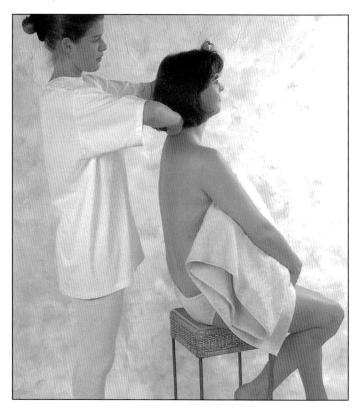

1 *Make sure your partner is comfortable and place your left hand over the forehead and the palm of your right hand across the back of the neck. Hold for a few moments and then release.*

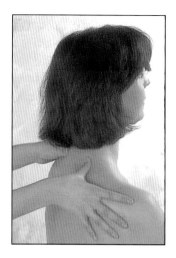

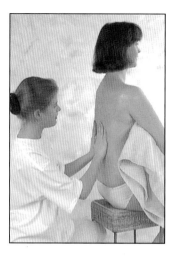

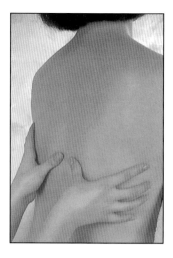

2 *Apply a little oil to your fingers and using a slight but gentle pressure, softly massage each side of your partner's neck and shoulders, kneading mainly with the thumbs. This will help to relieve the tension often caused by the weight of enlarged breasts.*

3 *Stroke the oil evenly over the back and begin an effleurage movement (a soothing, stroking motion with two hands, moving up the sides of the spine and out over the shoulders). Repeat several times to establish a rhythm and relax your partner.*

4 *Using the thumbs, work upward on each side of the spinal column from the lower back to the neck to help release congestion along the spinal nerves. Repeat four times. Clear the movement by sweeping up the back using the calming effleurage stroke.*

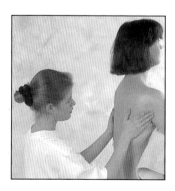

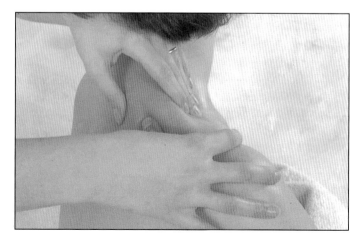

5 *Starting from the centre of the back, begin working up and outward across the width of the back with superficial effleurage movements. Repeat the movements several times until your partner is relaxed. This will help to stimulate the circulation and has a soothing effect on the nerve endings.*

6 *Using a double-handed movement, press down and then gently lift the muscles to the side of the neck, rolling with the thumb, and then release. Work out* *from the neck across the shoulder, and then repeat across the other shoulder. Performed slowly with rhythmic movements this is very relaxing and will alleviate stiffness.*

THE ABDOMEN

For a pregnant woman, the weight of the uterus can constrict important blood vessels if she lies down flat on her back, so provide plenty of pillows, cushions, bolsters or rolled towels to support your partner behind the back, under the neck and knees and anywhere else she needs to feel comfortable.

1 *Below: It may seem alarming to massage the abdomen during pregnancy but, providing the strokes are light and careful, it is safe and relaxing for mother and baby. Gentle massage all over the abdominal area can be very soothing and is beneficial for relieving the stretched feeling often experienced during pregnancy. Apply oil evenly over the area to help feed the tissues and lessen the possibility of stretch marks.*

2 *Using the flat of your hands, carefully glide them up from either side of the waist, lifting your hands off as they reach the navel, and then start again. Continue to stroke the area with a light, soft touch, working over the whole of the abdomen to soothe and calm.*

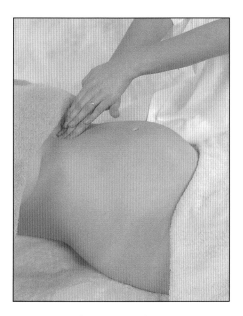

3 *After a minute of gentle circular movements, place the fingertips of your left hand on the higher section of the solar plexus region and cover with your right hand. Rest both hands for a moment and then release to help alleviate stress.*

LEGS

Make sure your partner is comfortable, with the knees supported by cushions.

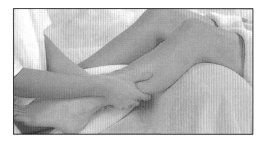

Begin gently stroking the leg with an effleurage from the ankle to the knee, smoothing up the shin and then glide around the calf.

It can help to relieve the swelling, varicose veins or cramp which afflict many pregnant women. Do not use any heavy movements to the legs and avoid any reflexology movements to the feet, though gentle stroking around the ankles may well be appreciated.

TO FINISH

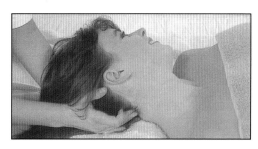

With both hands positioned at the back of the neck, apply light circular pressures to the cranium (skull) with your fingertips working in an upward direction to help release tension.

End the massage by smoothing the hair away from the neck and forehead, releasing all the negative energy. Allow your partner to rest for 15 minutes and then help her to get up very gently.

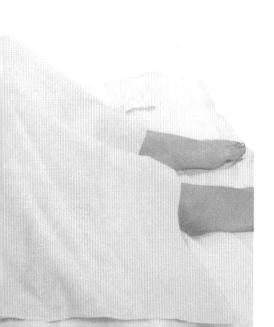

BEAUTY BASICS

Looking good starts with great skin, and aromatherapy can help you achieve this in various ways: the remarkable penetrative properties of essential oils make them excellent moisturizers, and the wide range of their properties means there is always the right oil for the right condition. For instance, rosemary stimulates the circulation and thyme help the cells to regenerate. As well as being stimulating to the lymphatic system, which helps cleanse the tissue that causes sluggish skin, essential oils can be used as part of your daily skin-care routine and to treat specific problems such as acne.

FEED YOUR SKIN

Skin needs to be fed and nourished – inside and out. Healthy diets can keep the body in shape but to keep skin in peak condition it needs to have a ready supply of valuable vitamins and minerals. Many factors can drain the body of this valuable resource – canned and over-processed foods, caffeine, alcohol, nicotine, sunlight, central heating, carbon monoxide and habitual drug taking. The effects of these can build up and attack the skin so from time to time you need to give it a break.

A one-day fruit and vegetable diet is an excellent regime to adopt once a month to cleanse your body and give a boost to your system.

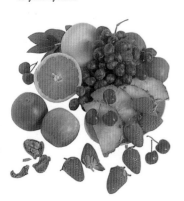

SKIN TYPES

Choose the right oils for your skin type and use them to blend your own cleansers, toners, masks and moisturizing facial oils. Remember that skin types can vary: skin may be drier in winter or summer or more prone to oiliness around the time of your period, and it can change several times between puberty and menopause. So review the oils you use to suit your skin now and vary them to meet the changing needs of your complexion.

Few people are blessed with normal skin and even those who are may tend towards dryness or oiliness at times. Letters in parentheses indicate what other skin types an oil is suitable for. D = dry, S = sensitive, O = oily, A = all skin types.

Oils for Normal Skin
Chamomile (D, S) · Fennel (O)
Geranium (A) · Lavender (A)
Lemon (O) · Patchouli (D)
Rose (D, S) · Sandalwood (D, S)

Oils for Dry Skin
Chamomile · Geranium · Lavender
Hyssop · Rose · Patchouli
Sandalwood · Ylang-Ylang

Oils for Sensitive Skin
Chamomile · Lavender · Neroli
Rose · Sandalwood

Oils for Oily Skin
Bergamot · Cedarwood · Cypress
Lavender · Lemon · Geranium
Juniper · Frankincense · Sage

Combination skin has an oily T-zone panel from the forehead down to the nose and chin area, and may be normal or dry elsewhere. Double up on the treatments, using oils for oily skin on the greasy patches and oils for normal skin on the rest of the face area.

CLEANSERS

Choose the correct essential oils for your skin type and blend them in with an ordinary unperfumed brand of cleanser, liquid soap, or tissue-off lotion/cream, and they will do nature's work of rebalancing the skin.

FACIAL STEAM

Add five drops of chamomile for a soothing steam or try lavender, peppermint, thyme or rosemary to stimulate; comfrey or fennel for their healing properties.

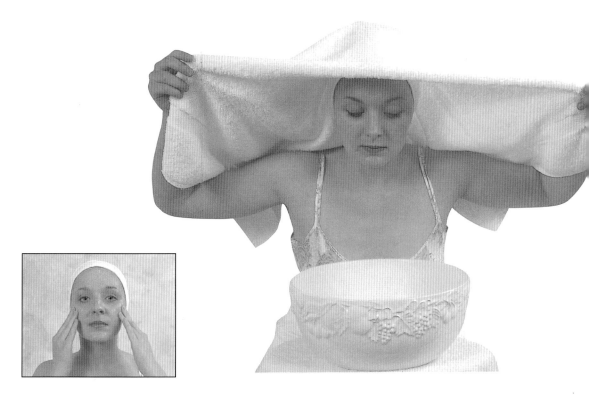

Above: Cleanse the face, paying particular attention to the oilier areas.

Above right: For a facial steam, boil the water, cool slightly and add the oils. Steam for five minutes.

Toners

Essential oils are the gentlest way of toning up. Rose water for normal or dry/sensitive skin or witchhazel for oilier skins are ideal bases for fresheners. These can be applied with cotton wool or for a more refreshing tone, sprayed on to the face.

Herbal tea infusions are also ideal toners. Boil a cup of water and infuse chamomile, marigold, rosehip or nettle teas (you can use herbal tea bags if you can't get hold of the herbs), add two drops of orange or lavender oil and leave

to cool. Oily skin benefits from juniper or lemongrass whereas drier skins would appreciate rose or sandalwood.

Facial Oils

Well-moisturized skin is soft and supple, reflects a healthy glow and ages less quickly. Younger skin only needs light conditioning whereas older skin needs specific nourishing treatments. Most moisturizers soothe and sit on the surface of the skin, but essential oils, with their fine molecular structure, work their way through from the surface to the inner dermis (the skin's deeper regenerating layer). Mixed with the correct amount of base oil, these pure essentials do not clog up pores on lubrication: they are light enough to be absorbed spontaneously by skin.

Use two tablespoons of base oil and add six drops of essential oil (maximum of three different oils) to suit individual needs.

Masks

Both clay and oatmeal are ideal ingredients for any face mask. A natural powdered clay is fuller's earth, which can be mixed into a paste with hot water. Cool and then add yogurt for a smoother consistency. Similarly, finely ground oatmeal can be mixed into a paste and left to cool. Add 15 drops of essential oils to suit your skin type per cupful of paste. Smooth on to your face, leave to dry slightly and then sponge off. For particularly dry/sensitive skins add one tablespoon evening primrose base oil to give a more moisturizing mask. When applying, avoid the eye area.

EYE TREATS

While relaxing with a face mask on, close the eyes and cover with cotton pads soaked in rose water, or soothe with two slices of fresh cucumber.

ACNE

Because of their anti-bacterial, anti-inflammatory and rebalancing properties, essential oils are ideal skin treatments for acne sufferers.

It is often a mistake to scrub oily skin over-zealously: this only activates the sebaceous glands which in turn produce more sebum. If you suffer from pustular acne then avoid excessive facial steams which may spread the condition: use a mask instead. Often it is better to opt for a daily sensitive-skin type cleanser and moisturizer, adding two drops of juniper, which is stimulating and antiseptic. Opt for a deeper clay-type mask treatment once a week, adding a couple of drops of juniper, which is healing, soothing and tightening, or eucalyptus which is anti-inflammatory, antiseptic and antibiotic. Increase your intake of vitamin E, which is a great skin healer.

BROKEN VEINS

These small, red, spider-like thread veins often appear on the surface of skin around the cheek area. They are broken capillaries and seem to affect those with a delicate or fragile skin type. Hot and cold elements, along with stimulants such as alcohol and caffeine, can often trigger this condition. To treat it at home the secret is to protect the skin from losing excess moisture and to give it extra essential oil treatments using parsley, geranium, chamomile, rosemary or cypress in a heavy base oil.

COLD SORES

Cold sores are small blisters on the lips or surrounding area which are caused by the virus herpes simplex. It normally lies dormant in nerve cells but can surface following a simple cold or flu. Any lip sore that persists should be treated medically but for the common cold sore a dab of undiluted tea tree oil will help.

ODD SPOTS

If prone to occasional spots then mix one drop each of neroli, lemon and lavender in one teaspoon (5 ml) of base oil and treat just the affected area. For a single spot use a cotton bud and dab on one drop of undiluted sandalwood.

FACIAL MASSAGE

Massage helps the skin to absorb oils and creams easily.
Give skin a clear start with our step-by-step facial.

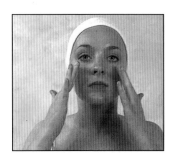

1 *Pour a small amount of blended oil into the palm of your hand and gently apply all over the face, avoiding the eyes.*

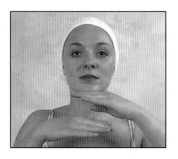

2 *With the back of your hands, gently tap the skin around the jaw-line and underneath the chin to stimulate the skin cells.*

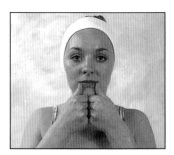

3 *Apply small circular movements to the chin area, using your thumbs, to tone, help circulation and eliminate toxins.*

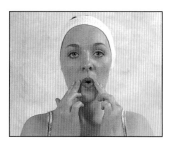

4 *Make an "oooh"-shaped mouth. Massage either side easing out fine lines.*

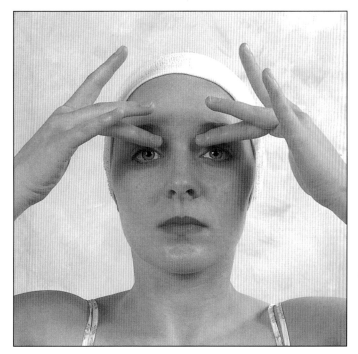

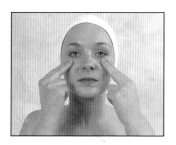

5 *With your fingertips, press along the top of the cheekbones and massage outward up to the temples to release toxins.*

6 *With the middle fingers, apply pressure to points above the bridge of the nose and underneath the eyebrows. Hold for five seconds*

and smooth across from the inner to the outer corners of the eyebrows and continue up to the temples.

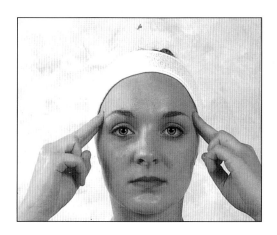

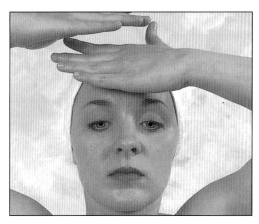

7 *To relieve tension, apply firm pressure at either side of the temples, and rotate backward.*

8 *Stroke up the forehead to the hairline with the palms of the hands, smoothing out fine lines.*

HEALTHY HAIR

Hair can define your image and style but it is also a mirror of your health. Emotional or physical problems can soon result in a lack of bounce or shine.

Keeping hair in peak condition is a combination of caring for it on the surface and nurturing it from inside with a well-balanced diet.

SCALP MASSAGE OILS

Dry hair is rough to touch, thick in texture and dries out at the first sign of heated rollers or tongs. Avoid chemical colourants and perms and opt for shampoos and conditioners with jojoba and almond oils. Hot oil treatments allow essential oils to soak in easily and condition the hair. After massaging warm oil into the scalp, wrap the head in a warm towel and leave on for half an hour.

Oils for Dry Hair
Rose · Sandalwood · Ylang-ylang
Lavender · Geranium

Greasy hair tends to look dull, lank, lacks body and won't hold a style. Central heating and environmental elements aggravate the condition but it can stem from a hormonal imbalance. Check your diet and avoid harsh degreasing shampoos. Clean brushes and combs weekly. Plastic brushes are better for brushing through as bristle continually stimulates the scalp. Choose light conditioning rinses to detangle but try a scalp massage to regulate the oil-producing sebaceous glands.

Oils for Greasy Hair
Basil · Eucalyptus · Cedarwood
Chamomile · Lemongrass
Cypress · Sage · Rosemary

Normal hair is glossy with plenty of natural body and bounce. An occasional hot-oil scalp treatment

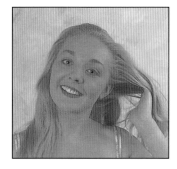

will keep it looking good and growing healthily.

Oils for Normal Hair
Geranium · Lavender
Lemongrass · Rosemary

Combination hair has ends that are dry or normal and the roots are greasy. Avoid using hot appliances near the scalp and keep the ends regularly trimmed and conditioned. Use a scalp treatment with oils for greasy hair but don't comb through to the ends.

How to Mix
Base oils Choose from sweet almond, apricot kernal, avocado, jojoba, evening primrose or sunflower.

Essential oils For one scalp treatment, choose up to three oils and use five drops of each for two tablespoons of base oil (for very long hair you may need more oil). Warm the blended oils by placing the container in a bowl of boiling

water, and then massage into the scalp. Wrap with a hot towel, leave for 15 minutes and then shampoo.

HAIR PROBLEMS

Dandruff
There are two types: dry and the more common oily. It's not catching! It can be caused by factors such as chemical body changes, stress, poor eating habits or wrong application of hair products. Both flakey and dry scalps can be treated with essential oils. Use special dandruff shampoos and conditioning rinses and treat the scalp by gently massaging with oils to suit. Use a base oil formula with patchouli and tea tree. For a dry, itchy scalp try cedarwood and lavender.

Grey Hair
Grey hair is more porous and needs extra conditioning, particularly if it is chemically treated or coloured. Use a scalp formula for dry hair adding essential oil enhancers like chamomile to lighten or sage to darken any discolouration.

Hair Loss
Hair coming out in handfuls is often due to a hormonal imbalance, stress or anxiety, so the first step is to learn to relax. Any unusual thinning patch should be looked at by a trichologist but, as a general remedy, use a scalp massage with lavender and rosemary oils.

SCALP MASSAGE

This is a wonderful way to condition hair, stimulate the scalp and relieve tension. You can use these steps to treat your own hair but it's even more relaxing if you can persuade a friend to help, especially if you've got long hair.

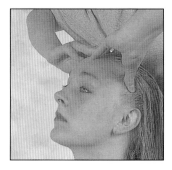

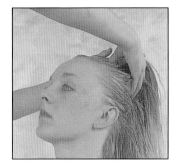

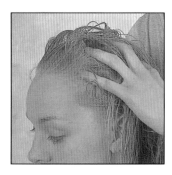

1 *Shampoo the hair and towel dry to absorb excess water. Comb through with a wide-tooth comb. Tilt your head back and pour some oil on to the hairline, massaging in with thumbs on the temple and fingers spread apart over the centre of the head.*

2 *Loosely run fingers and oil over the top of the scalp from front to back, lifting hair at the crown. Keep dipping your fingertips in the treatment oil to spread through the hair while massaging.*

3 *Massage the head with kneading movements. Grip and push (with fingerpads, rather than fingernails) against the scalp. The scalp should gently rotate against the skull. Concentrate on one area at a time, with the hands positioned on either side of the scalp.*

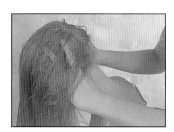

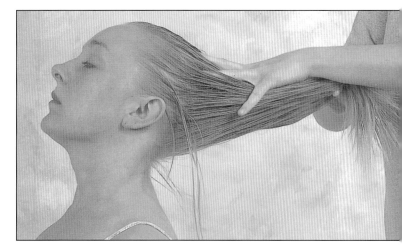

4 *Scalp massage works from front to back, from the forehead, frontal hairline, temples and sides, over the crown of the head to the base of the neck, following the natural flow of blood. If the scalp feels particularly tight then concentrate on areas where the scalp doesn't want to move. At the base of the skull, press firmly and push the whole scalp up toward the crown to release tension.*

5 *Pull any extra oil through the hair, working out from the roots to the tips. Make sure all the* hair is well oiled, and then leave towel-wrapped for at least 15 minutes before shampooing.

THE AROMATIC BATH

The relaxing and remedial properties of water and of massaging oils into the body were recognized in ancient Greek and Roman cultures, when bathing first became a daily ritual.

A bath with essential oils is one of the simplest and most effective aromatherapy treatments. It can be stimulating or relaxing, depending on the temperature of the water and whether you choose oils with uplifting or calming properties. In the bath, the therapeutic action of the oils is two-fold: they are absorbed through the skin, moisturizing the dermis and entering the circulatory system, and at the same time their aromas are inhaled, stimulating the brain and increasing your sense of well-being. An aromatic bath can detoxify the body, help problems like cellulite, joint stiffness, general aches and pains, colds and headaches, tone and condition skin, and relieve anxiety and tension.

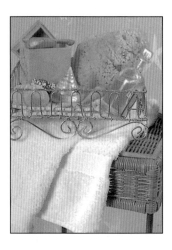

RUNNING THE BATH

Bath temperature and the time spent in the tub are important. A cooler bath is more stimulating and warmer water relaxes. Very hot water is damaging, however: it causes blood vessels and capillaries to expand and increases the heart beat. You should particularly avoid hot water if you have varicose veins, haemorrhoids, high blood pressure or are pregnant. A 15–20 minute soak is long enough before skin cells over-hydrate and swell with water. Wait until the bath is almost full before adding the oils, as they evaporate so quickly.

OILS FOR THE BATH

Essential oils are the best way of making a bath both aromatic and therapeutic. They sink into the skin easily and at the same time impart their lovely herbal or floral fragrances. You can add drops of oil directly to the bath and they will float on the surface in a fine film and evaporate, giving you the full benefit of their aromas. Or if you want to absorb them more you can disperse them through the water by mixing with a base carrier oil such as sweet almond, apricot kernel, jojoba or evening primrose (these rich base oils all nourish and rejuvenate the skin in their own right).

Mix a bath oil with a combination of up to three essential oils, five drops from each, in one tablespoon of skin-softening base oil. Choose oils with similar or complementary effects so they do not counter-balance one another.

THE RELAXING BATH

To calm yourself after a fraught day or to prepare yourself for a peaceful night's sleep, turn your bathroom into a private sanctuary. Keep the light soft if possible, or use an eye mask or burn aromatic candles. Plants create an oxygenated atmosphere. Support your head with a bath pillow, close your eyes and inhale deeply. Concentrate on your breathing, empty your mind and let the oils soothe away the stresses and strains. After a 15–20 minute soak, get out slowly and wrap yourself in a large, warm towel.

Oils for Relaxation
Basil · Bergamot · Cedarwood Chamomile · Frankincense Hyssop · Juniper · Lavender Marjoram · Melissa · Neroli Patchouli · Rose · Sage Sandalwood · Ylang-Ylang

Although these oils have a predominantly calming effect some can also be used to stimulate the circulation and lymphatic system, in particular lavender oil and also bergamot.

THE STIMULATING BATH

Best for the morning to get you started or to revive you before an evening out. Keep the water fairly cool and use an invigorating bath mitt to rub down and stimulate the circulation. When you've soaked, rinse yourself with water as cold as you can bear, either by splashing directly from the tap (faucet) or shower, or by adding more cold water to cool down your bath.

As you get out, either slap yourself dry to make the skin tingle or rub yourself vigorously with a towel.

Oils for Stimulation
Cypress · Eucalyptus · Fennel
Geranium · Juniper · Lavender
Lemon · Lemongrass · Peppermint
Pine · Rosemary · Thyme

THERAPEUTIC BATHS

Oils for Dermatitis
Chamomile · Hyssop · Lavender
Oils for Eczema
Chamomile · Geranium · Hyssop
Juniper · Rosemary · Myrrh
Oils for Psoriasis
Bergamot · Chamomile · Lavender
Oils for Arthritis/Rheumatism
Chamomile · Eucalyptus · Juniper
Lavender · Rosemary · Thyme

SHOWERS AND COLD RINSES

nvigorating jets of water are ideal for getting the blood pumping and there's no need to forego the benefits of aromatic oils. Skin tends to be sluggish in the cold winter months but sloughing off dead top layers can help regenerate cells and allow moisturizers to be absorbed more easily. Showers are ideal for smoothing skin with exfoliating rubs using wet salt, a loofah or a mitt to slough off the top surface of dead skin cells. A dry friction glove or loofah is too harsh for most skins so soften first in warm water. Soft bristle brushes can also help to get the circulation going with gentle massage on problem areas like hips and thighs. To keep friction brushes and mitts fresh always rinse and hang up to dry.

Essential oils can be used under the shower: try a base oil mixed with invigorating essences and with a clean face-cloth or sponge, pour on the oils and rub all over the body in circular motions whilst showering. To clear the sinuses and help coughs and colds, sponge the chest with a mix of eucalyptus and peppermint oils. A cold-water shower after cleansing improves the circulation and tightens skin pores.

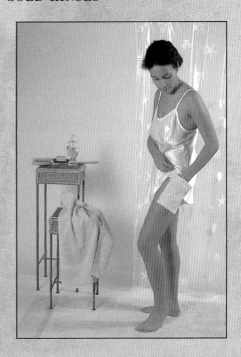

Start off your shower or bath routine by whisking off dead skin cells with a friction mitt. Moisten the palm of the mitt with warm water or softening oils such as sweet almond or evening primrose. Concentrate on outer thighs, working from the knee in upward circular movements across the buttocks.

AFTER-BATH BODY TREATMENTS

Moisturizing oils and lotions applied after the bath or shower help to nourish the skin, keeping it soft and supple. As we get older our skin dehydrates since the oil glands do not produce as much oil as in youth.

Apply a body oil all over the body, starting from the feet and working right up to the neck and tips of the ears. Avoid talcum powders which clog the pores and tend to have a drying effect.

BODY-OIL FORMULA

Essential oils sink beautifully into warm damp skin. For a lasting effect, mix the three chosen bath essential oils, five drops of each, in two tablespoons of base oil. If you want to make up a larger quantity of body oil, use a concentration of three per cent essential oil in base oil.

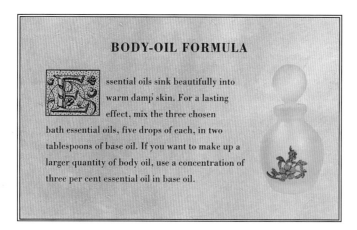

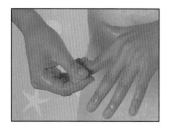

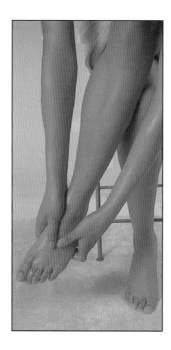

Above: Condition hands and nails with a simple finger-pulling exercise. Spread and stretch the fingers straight out; massage each finger with oils, working from the tip of the nails to the cuticles and up to each finger knuckle.

Right: Soften the feet after a bath by massaging between the toes and then working around the tougher skin and heel areas. Finish with sweeping movements all over to stimulate the circulation.

PROBLEM ZONES

Hands and nails take some rough treatment with everyday chores. The ideal time for a manicure or pedicure is after soaking in a bath when nails and skin are softened, making it easy to clean around the nail bed and to clip uneven nails without snagging.

Fragile or flakey nails benefit from a rich, nourishing treatment: rub them with apricot kernel, wheatgerm or jojoba oil. Restore hands with a soothing, moisturizing mix of one tablespoon of sweet almond oil and five drops each of patchouli, lavender and lemon.

Feet are often neglected until they hurt. Polish hard skin around heels and soles with a handful of damp salt or use a pumice stone. While in the bath, bend one knee, grip the toes and then work with the fingers massaging in an upward direction, from the toes to the heels and up the calves in order to stimulate blood flow and relax tired feet. Massage a body oil into the feet after a bath, shower or pedicure.

For a deodorizing and soothing footbath add three drops each of cypress and lavender to a basin full of water. Chilblains can be treated with a massage blend of three drops of geranium and a drop each of lavender and rosemary in one tablespoon of sweet almond base oil.

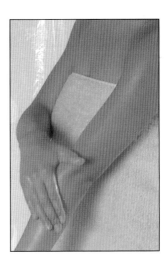

Above: Apply body oil to the arms with smooth upward strokes, concentrating on the elbows and upper arms where the skin is often rougher and drier.

Elbows can soon build up hard protective layers of grey, unsightly skin. A good softener for tough elbows is a sweet almond oil and oatmeal scrub. Mix three tablespoons of sweet almond oil with three tablespoons of fine oatmeal and mix to a paste with fresh milk or yoghurt. Smooth and rub over the elbows and any grey, goosey areas of skin around upper arms. Add six drops of fennel if arms are flabby. Another great elbow booster is the traditional recipe of cutting a lemon in half, squeezing out the juice and rubbing the elbows in the hollow of the lemon.

Left: When it comes to applying body oil, the back, neck and shoulders are often neglected because they are difficult to reach, but these are key areas for releasing tension and the skin needs to be nourished, so smooth as far as possible, or enlist the help of a friend.

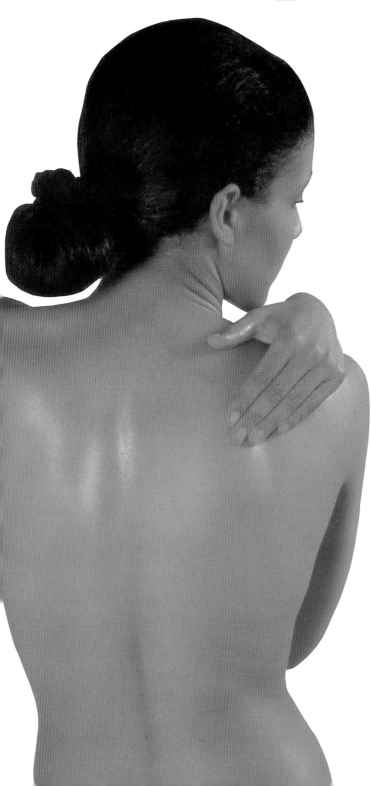

IN THE REALM OF THE SENSES

The power of perfume to inspire romance has been known since the Babylonians, and perfume and flowers are still today the favourite gifts for lovers. Cleopatra's seduction of Mark Antony was carefully staged with a carpet of rose petals and rare and exotic scents in every conceivable form – even the sails of her barge were drenched in perfume to catch the breeze and announce her arrival.

The sense of smell is fundamental to our sensuality. Pheromones, chemicals secreted in human sweat, act as the most basic trigger to sexual attraction. The smells of flowers and plants are the plant equivalent of pheromones, irresistible to birds and bees and just as attractive to humans. We can use natural aromatic plant oils to relax, heighten our awareness, excite the senses and create a mood for love.

SETTING THE SCENE

Create a calming and sensual atmosphere with scented candles or a few drops of essential oil evaporated in a fragrancer or light-bulb ring. Dim the lights and turn up the heat.

Scent your lingerie or bedlinen by adding three drops of your favourite oil to the final rinse, or store them in drawers with aromatic bags or scented balls. Sprinkle drops of rose or jasmine on the pillows.

PREPARING YOUR BODY

Luxuriate in an aromatic bath or hot tub, or, better still, share it with your partner. After soaking, perfume your whole body with a rich body oil or use a strong concentration to dab pulse points such as wrists, temples and behind the ears and knees, and wait for your partner to discover these secret scented areas.

PARTNER MASSAGE

We are all sensual beings and yet at times we may need help to switch off from everyday concerns and tune in to our senses. The loving touch of partner massage is always enjoyable; it is relaxing and yet sensually stimulating – a total physical experience.

You can adapt the basic essential massage, using plenty of *effleurage* all over, deeper kneading for tense areas and light feather strokes with the fingertips to excite the surface of the skin. Avoid the lymph drainage movements as these are distinctly unerotic! Discover your partner's erogenous zones – explore the ears and feet and the inside of the forearms and thighs. Find some more. Be tender and loving, playful and creative – let your imagination guide you.

OILS FOR SEDUCTION

Most of the aphrodisiac oils combine well with each other, but be careful not to use too many together or they may clash and work against each other. Subtlety is the key to the art of seduction.

● *Clary sage* – sweet, sensuous and slightly intoxicating, but be careful as in high doses its sedative effect will inhibit sex drive.
● *Geranium* – a strong floral that both relaxes and uplifts.
● *Jasmine* – the heady floral fragrance boosts confidence and creates a luxurious atmosphere.
● *Neroli* – fresh and sweet, its fortifying effect helps overcome shyness and inhibitions.
● *Patchouli* – heavy and exotic, it is stimulating in small doses and heightens the senses.
● *Rose* – the quintessential oil for lovers. Rare and powerful.
● *Sandalwood* – woody, sweet and exotic with spicy undertones.
● *Ylang-Ylang* – the long-lasting floral scent gives a feeling of relaxed well-being, helpful for impotence or frigidity.

You can also try the warm, spicy exotics such as black pepper, ginger, cardamon, cinnamon or cedarwood, but be sparing with these as they can easily overpower.

Layer the scents by choosing just three or four and using them in different strengths and combinations for the room fragrance, bath, body oil or massage blend.

With a massage oil blended from floral and spicy aphrodisiac essences you can arouse the intimate senses of touch and smell simultaneously as you explore the skin and curves of your partner's body with strong smoothing strokes. Let the heady scents work their spell on the senses and emotions.

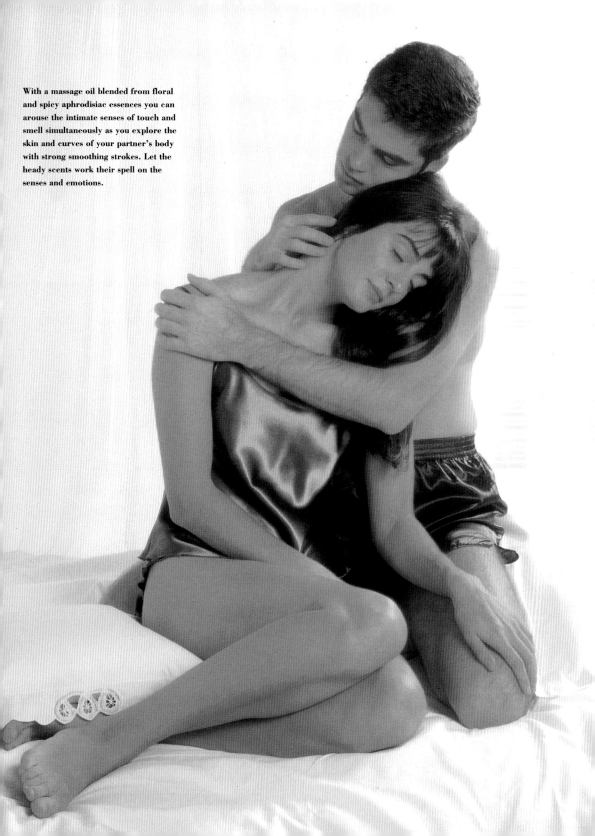

AMBIENT AROMAS

A lingering smell, whether pleasant or foul, is usually the first thing we notice when we enter a room, and it can strongly affect the way we feel. Fragrancing the home to cover unpleasant smells and delight the senses is an old tradition. For centuries the Chinese have suspended balls of jasmine flowers over the bed to clear the air and promote pleasant dreams, while posies of jasmine were handed to guests to refresh them on leaving banquets or dances. Lavender sachets placed in drawers and bowls of pot pourri to scent a room were particular favourites of the Victorians.

STUDIES AND OFFICES

Work-places are often stuffy and full of unpleasant smells, but if you work in an open-plan space fragrancing the whole area may not be a viable option. Inhaling a few drops of oil from a handkerchief is the most personal way of using a fragrance, or you can spray your immediate environment with a room spray, or add a couple of drops of oil to a cup of hot water on your desk.

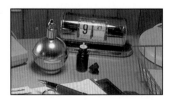

Useful oils for the work-place are basil, rosemary, bergamot, lemon and melissa. Bergamot and lemon are particularly antiseptic, and lemon has the added advantage of helping efficiency. Basil stimulates a tired brain and rosemary is a great aid to concentration. Rosemary is also helpful in relieving headaches. If you are feeling overwrought try clary sage or juniper, but watch the dosage as too much will cause sleepiness.

LIVING ROOMS

The methods for fragrancing a room are many and diverse. Those that involve evaporating the oils, such as fragrancers/diffusers, water bowls, light-bulb rings and room sprays, are best for preventing ill-health, balancing the emotions and disguising unpleasant smells such as cigarette smoke or cooking odours. All these methods disperse the fragrance through a large space extremely quickly and effectively. For more lingering and subtle scents, blend your own pot pourri or, alternatively, use pomanders.

Rose, geranium, orange and lavender are pleasing and uplifting scents for a room, used individually or blended together.

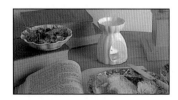

For an exotic, intimate atmosphere use sandalwood or patchouli, or to unwind in the evening try geranium, lavender, sandalwood or ylang-ylang.

Perfumes for parties

Clary sage or jasmine will create a heady, "feel-good" atmosphere for a party, or use orange, lemongrass or neroli for a lighter, fresher touch.

For a festive blend choose from the spicier oils such as frankincense, cedarwood, sandalwood, cinnamon and orange.

BEDROOMS

Whether to ensure a restful night's sleep or to turn your bedroom into a place of passion, fragrancing the bedroom just before retiring will create an appropriate atmosphere. Rose, neroli and lavender are delightful all-purpose oils for the bedroom. Use lavender to freshen a musty spare room to make it welcoming for guests.

INSECT REPELLANT

Use tea tree, eucalyptus, melissa, lemon grass or the closely related citronella in a diffuser to keep insects at bay.

DISINFECTING

Vaporized molecules of any essential oil will neutralize airborne bacteria, but some – such as tea tree, bergamot, lemon, pine and lavender – are particularly antiseptic. Use these in a fragrancer or room spray. Pine, lemon and tea tree can be used on a damp cloth to disinfect surfaces in the kitchen or bathroom. Clear the atmosphere of a sickroom with bergamot, eucalyptus and juniper.

POT POURRI

To make your own pot pourri assemble fully-dried flowers, petals, herbs, leaves and other plant materials. There are no hard and fast rules about quantities and proportions, but an allowance of two or three tablespoons ground spices, two tablespoons orris-root powder, two teaspoons dried lemon, orange or lime peel, and six drops of essential oil to every four cups of dried plant material makes a pleasant balanced mixture.

If your pot pourri loses a little of its aroma over a period of time, it can be revived. Simply stir in another two or three drops of essential oil. And if the mixture loses its colour sharpness just stir in a few dried flowers such as miniature rosebuds, santolina flowers or tansy clusters.

Cottage Garden Mix

1 cup dried lavender flowers
1 cup dried rose petals
1 cup dried pinks (*Dianthus*)
1 cup dried scented geranium
  leaves
1 tbsp (15g) ground cinnamon
2 tsp (10g) ground allspice
1 tsp (5g) dried grated lemon peel
2 tbsp (30g) orris-root powder
3 drops rose oil
3 drops geranium oil
Mix ingredients together in a covered container, and set aside for six weeks. Stir daily to distribute the fragrances.

Woodland Mix

1 cup lime seedpods, or "keys"
1 cup cedar bark shavings
1 cup sandalwood shavings
1 cup small cones
1 tbsp (15g) whole cloves
1 tbsp (15g) star anise
1 stick cinnamon, crushed
2 tbsp (30g) orris-root powder
4 drops sandalwood oil
2 drops cinnamon oil
Mix ingredients together in a covered container and set aside for six weeks. Stir daily.

Ingredients which can be used to make pot pourri. From the left: dried rosemary, lavender, and bay leaves, dried ground orris-root powder, dried rosemary leaves, a selection of essential oils, ground cinnamon, dried chilies and cinnamon sticks, whole cloves, a blend of dried flowers, limes and lemons. The dried peel of citrus fruit is finely grated or chopped for use in the spice mixture.

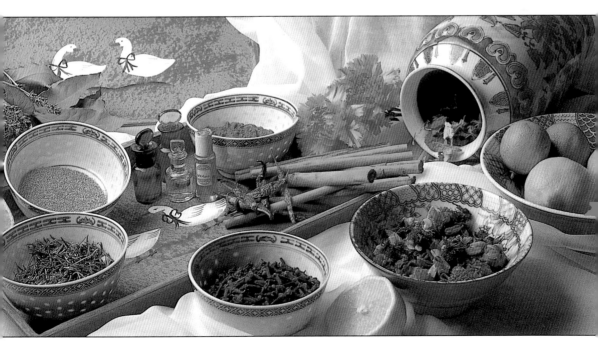

THE STRESS FACTOR

Pressure can be stimulating, challenging and motivating, but if it builds up we may be left feeling unable to cope. Our response is often to deny the pressure and ignore the physical signs of stress such as fatigue, self-doubt, sleeplessness and headaches. If the symptoms and causes of stress are left untreated they will affect your general health and well-being, and can even lead to serious illness, such as ulcers, heart attacks and clinical depression, so it's important to start tackling problems at an early stage, before they erupt. De-stressing requires a positive tactical plan for learning how to cope and retain a balanced outlook on life.

Aromatherapy is a marvellous antidote to many of the problems associated with stress as it draws on the calming, relaxing, uplifting and restorative powers of particular essential oils, providing a natural and powerful alternative to tranquillizers, anti-depressants and other drugs. They can work to relax the nervous system and give it enough stimulation to rebalance and control itself, leaving you refreshed and ready to cope.

ANXIETY

Whether it's a temporary bout of nerves, caused by something like an impending examination or interview, or an ongoing response to a persistent problem, anxiety can be a debilitating response to stress. It prevents you from dealing effectively with a problem and makes you feel tense. Essential oils, when inhaled, stimulate the lymbic portion of the brain which is responsible for all our feelings of well-being and discontent. They can balance the senses before deep depression sets into a more serious state. Temporary anxiety can also trigger skin eruptions so watch your diet and boost levels of vitamins C and E and B-complex.

Anxiety can be alleviated with a combination of uplifting and calming oils.

Basil (uplifting) · Bergamot (uplifting) · Geranium (relaxing) Lavender (soothing) · Neroli (sedative) · Sandalwood (calming)

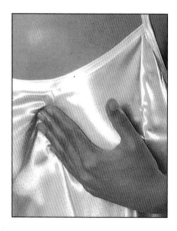

SOLAR PLEXUS STROKE

A marvellous way of unlocking tension by calming the main nerves that run through this area. Use your left hand (for calming) to stroke the solar plexus (located just below the breast bone) in anti-clockwise circles. Close your eyes as you do this and try to empty your mind. It can help soothe you even if you're clothed, but the effect is enhanced if you use a relaxing oil such as lavender or geranium. Try it while your bath is running, or when lying in bed before you go to sleep.

You can use the oils individually or mix them, using two relaxing oils to one uplifting oil. A good combination is basil, neroli and lavender. Stick to the same blend and proportions for bath and body, mixing five drops of each of the three oils in one tablespoon of base oil for the bath and two tablespoons for the body. All of the oils can be used individually in light-ring burners or fragrancers.

MILD SHOCK

This is a temporary form of stress, but the impact on the system can nonetheless be very strong, so a fast-acting remedy is needed.

Chamomile (calming) · Rosemary (stimulating) · Melissa (anti-depressant) · Neroli (relieves anxiety) · Peppermint (invigorating pain-reliever)

Use only two essential oils: both camphor and melissa work well individually with neroli, and peppermint has an affinity with melissa. Use a total of six drops in

$1^1/_2$ tablespoons of base oils, with smaller quantities of rosemary (for example, four drops of rosemary to six drops of melissa). For fast relief add four drops to a handkerchief and inhale.

HEADACHES

Often one of the first signs of stress and a regular affliction for many people. Cold compresses of lavender or geranium across the forehead provide pleasant relief. Add five drops of one oil to a small bowl of cool or warm water, soak a cloth in the water, wring out and lay it across the forehead. To help a headache caused by tension in the neck, try a sandalwood compress across the neck. Scalp massage is soothing, or try the shiatsu headache relief steps.

DEPRESSION

The blues can hit us all from time to time, as financial, emotional or work problems hang over like a dark cloud. In the long term, if problems are not resolved, depression lowers the immune system, leaving you prone to a spiral of worsening mental and physical health. Essential oils can work wonders in lifting the spirits to prevent this.

Uplifting Oils
Bergamot · Cypress · Lemongrass Rosemary · Sage

Soothing Oils
Chamomile · Geranium · Jasmine Lavender · Marjoram · Neroli Patchouli · Rose · Sandalwood Ylang-Ylang

Start off with three soothing oils, and then drop one of these in favour of an uplifting oil to give an element of stimulation, and eventually introduce two

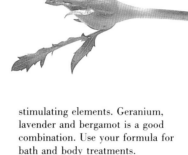

stimulating elements. Geranium, lavender and bergamot is a good combination. Use your formula for bath and body treatments.

Depression can be difficult to lift and if it persists you should consult a doctor or mental-health professional.

MENTAL FATIGUE

When you feel near to exhaustion or cannot concentrate on one thing at a time because problems seem to be crowding in on you, listen to your body's warning signals. Take time to unwind (try a bath with any of the soothing oils listed for depression), clear your head with a walk or deep-breathing exercises, and then revive yourself with oils such as eucalyptus and peppermint. Rosemary is helpful in concentrating the mind and stimulating the body so that you can continue to work if you feel you really can't afford to take a break.

INSOMNIA

Sleeplessness is a common response to stress, as your mind and body refuse to let go enough to give you the rest that you need. Learning to relax has to be built into a daily pattern with a healthy diet, regular exercise, and a calming routine to wind down before bedtime. Try a milky drink or herbal tea last thing at night. Have a relaxing bath and massage, drawing on the sedative powers of up to three of the following oils:

Chamomile · Cedarwood Frankincense · Hyssop · Lavender Marjoram · Melissa · Neroli Orange · Patchouli · Rose · Sage Sandalwood · Ylang-Ylang

Breathing aromatic vapours in the bedroom helps to induce sleep: *Frankincense* is warming and relaxing, and encourages tranquillity. Use in a fragrancer. *Lavender*'s relaxing quality can be harnessed by dabbing two drops on the edge of your pillow. *Marjoram* has excellent soporific properties. Release in a light-bulb ring or fragrancer. *Neroli*'s wonderful floral fragrance is also sedative. Two drops on the pillow or in a fragrancer will help disperse unpleasant thoughts.

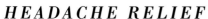

HEADACHE RELIEF

Headaches and migraines are common symptoms of stress. Follow these simple shiatsu steps to sweep away the tension, relieve pain and clear the head. The sequence is quick and easy to administer; it can be used anywhere and friends and colleagues will be grateful for the relief of their pain. You can perform some of the steps on yourself, though the healing touch of another's hands is more effective.

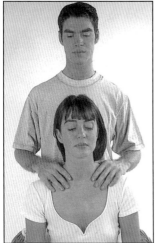

1 *Establish communication with your partner by placing both hands loosely on either side of the neck. Gently massage the shoulders; this helps to relax the breathing and creates a feeling of well-being.*

2 *Right: Tilt the head to the side and support with the palm of the hand so that the neck muscles can relax. Place the forearm across the shoulder and apply gentle downward pressure; hold for 5–10 seconds and then repeat with the other side. This movement is particularly good for opening the meridians running along the shoulders and neck.*

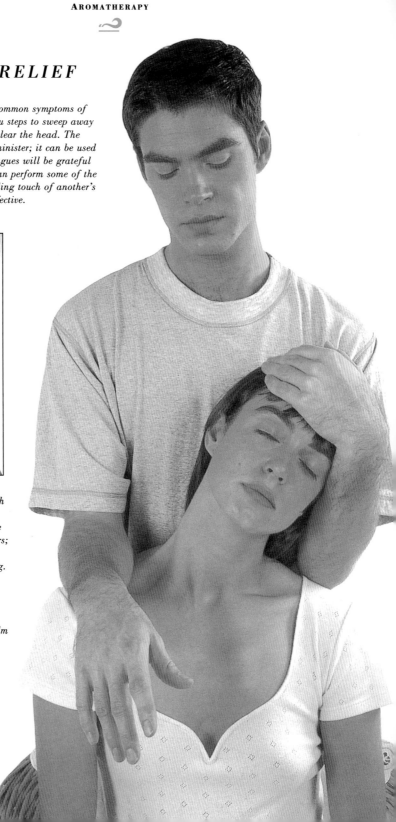

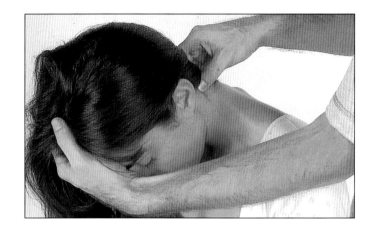

3 *Supporting the head with the left hand, work with thumb and forefinger applying gentle pressure from the base of the neck to the nape. Hold at the nape of the neck for five seconds and then release the built-up tension.*

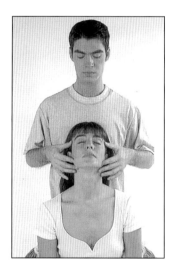

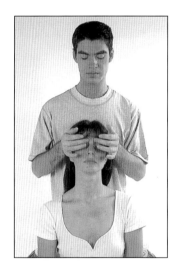

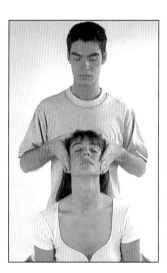

4 *Tilt the head back slightly, supporting it on your chest. Place your thumbs on the temples with the fingers loosely resting on either side of face. Gently rotate the thumbs in small forward movements.*

5 *Find the pressure points just above the inner corner of each eye. Apply gentle pressure with the middle fingers to help disperse the pain. Hold the pressure points for five seconds.*

6 *Position your thumbs on either side of the head just above the hairline – approximately two inches (5 cm) apart – with palms pressed flat along the sides of the face. Press the thumbs evenly back along the top of the head. This is a sensitive but invigorating movement to end the treatment.*

A shiatsu treatment is usually very effective for relieving stress and headaches but if your headache persists, consult a doctor. Avoid the treatment during pregnancy.

LEARNING TO RELAX

Relaxation is a prescription for health. Along with a well-balanced diet, an exercise programme, and a positive attitude towards recognizing and coping with stress, relaxation will help you balance the body and mind, even when you're worried and under pressure.

Exercise combats stress. The physically fitter you are, the better the body and mind can cope. Even burning off steam without losing self-control can be beneficial: a competitive racket sport, thumping the pillow, or going for a long walk can all release built-up tensions. Times of stress and emotional upset can make the body cry out for certain foods. Resist chocolate, cakes, ice cream or addictive stimulants like caffeine or nicotine. Feed the mind with a high intake of vitamin C from fresh fruit and vegetables, in particular citrus, berry and tropical fruits, and all of the B-complex vitamins.

WHOLE-BODY RELAXATION

Lie down straight with shoulders relaxed and even on the floor. Arms should be straight with elbows alongside the waist, palms turned upward. Relax your head and close the eyes. Breathe in deeply; allow your body to sink into the floor. Breathe out slowly; relax. Focus attention on your breathing; listen as you inhale and exhale and see how quiet the deep breathing can become.

Focus on breathing in and out, slowly and evenly.

Feet slightly apart and allowed to roll out naturally.

Let go of any tension in the knees.

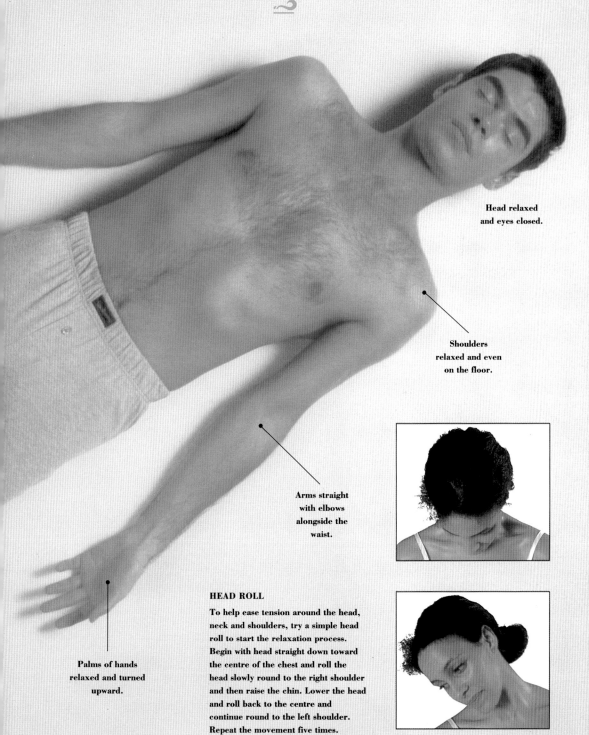

Head relaxed
and eyes closed.

Shoulders
relaxed and even
on the floor.

Arms straight
with elbows
alongside the
waist.

Palms of hands
relaxed and turned
upward.

HEAD ROLL

To help ease tension around the head,
neck and shoulders, try a simple head
roll to start the relaxation process.
Begin with head straight down toward
the centre of the chest and roll the
head slowly round to the right shoulder
and then raise the chin. Lower the head
and roll back to the centre and
continue round to the left shoulder.
Repeat the movement five times.

83

SHIATSU

The roots of shiatsu can be traced back over 5000 years to the ancient Chinese forms of medicine such as acupuncture and acupressure. However, it is a modern Japanese therapy, which fuses traditional Eastern practices with Western techniques of osteopathy. Literally translated the name means finger pressure – *Shi* (finger) and *Atsu* (pressure), although elbows, knees and feet are also used to press along the body's network of meridian lines and pressure points, releasing blocked channels of energy. It is an holistic method of alleviating pain and promoting health in the whole body.

SHIATSU MERIDIANS

Shiatsu is a manipulative therapy which uses static pressure applied to specific points and lines all over the body. The lines along which many of the points are situated are known as meridians. These meridian lines, which have been described as "channels of living magnetic energy", flow throughout the body and connect the main vital organs. It is this vital energy, known as "*Ki*", which keeps our bodies active, and the quality of our *Ki* depends upon our mental, emotional, physical and spiritual conditions.

An imbalance in a person's vital energy levels may manifest itself as a back problem, headache, or in many other ways. By working along the meridians, the therapist summons energy to the place most vulnerable and disperses the trapped energy from the areas where it is congested, thus restoring balance to the whole body.

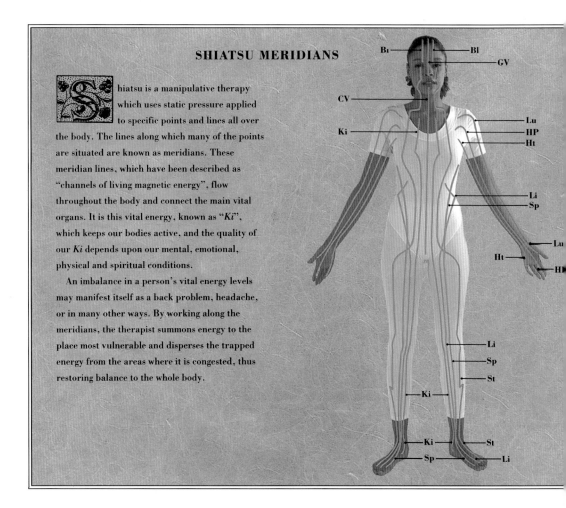

GIVING A SHIATSU SESSION

If your partner closes their eyes, this can make the session a special time to relax and switch off the world. There is no need to talk during a treatment as the communication of touch can say so much more. One of the fundamental principles of shiatsu is to have simultaneous touch from both hands. With a two-hand connection a circuit is created, bonding the giver and receiver. To keep this link, one hand is stationary – the support hand – and plays the role of listening and comforting your partner, while the other hand – the messenger hand – moves and does all the work. The amount of pressure from both hands will vary with the area of the body you are working on. The messenger and support hands change roles many times throughout a session. What you are trying to achieve is two points of contact merging and feeling like one to both therapist and partner.

Even as a beginner use your senses of looking, asking, listening and touching. Listen to your partner's needs and ask about symptoms before giving a treatment. Your motivation to help can be felt by your partner through the hands, transforming the simplest techniques into a caring bond. Before giving a shiatsu treatment, calm the mind, as any tension will transmit itself to your partner.

The Hara
The *Hara* is one of the most powerful energy centres of the body. In shiatsu terms it is known as the *Tanden*, and is located below the navel in the lower abdomen. It is the physical centre of the body and features prominently in all shiatsu treatments. The *Hara* incorporates the *Yin* (Earth) force flowing up the front of the body, and the *Yang* (Heaven) force flowing down the back merging into the lower abdomen. By focusing all movements from this centre, you can give harmonious and supportive treatments. Develop an open-posture principle in which your *Hara* is physically and energetically behind all your movements. This enables weight to be used instead of force. The simple rule is if you're not feeling comfortable and relaxed your partner will become aware of this.

Breathing is very important when stretching and applying pressure. Breathe in deeply and exhale as you move into a stretch, encouraging your partner to do the same.

Healing Energy
The aim of shiatsu is to balance the body's "*Ki*" energy levels. The rocking, kneading and stretching techniques are most effective in unblocking the congested areas. If your partner has a low energy

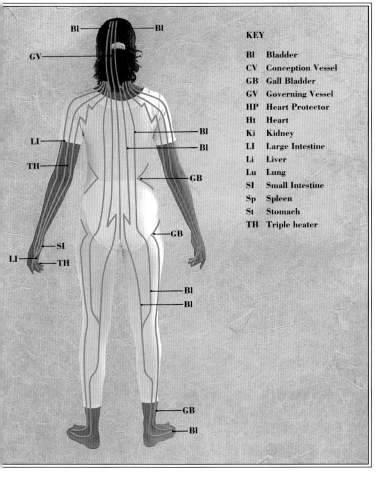

KEY

Bl	Bladder
CV	Conception Vessel
GB	Gall Bladder
GV	Governing Vessel
HP	Heart Protector
Ht	Heart
Ki	Kidney
LI	Large Intestine
Li	Liver
Lu	Lung
SI	Small Intestine
Sp	Spleen
St	Stomach
TH	Triple heater

level, and is generally fatigued, then slow, deep, static and perpendicular pressure will be more effective in strengthening the energy flow. Holding certain points from one to ten seconds is a general guideline but use your intuition as to how long you hold.

Practical Points

A shiatsu session normally lasts up to an hour. It is advisable to wear loose clothing so that your movements aren't hampered. The receiver is also clothed, but avoid bulky or constricting clothes that would impede contact with the body. Generally, the therapist works on the whole of the body and having discovered your problems may suggest simple practical exercises for home use to help the process of recovery. The effects of shiatsu may be felt immediately or later on in the same day, but if painful reactions are later experienced then your practitioner should be contacted. There are no two people with similar mental and physical complaints and the number of sessions will depend upon the individual's needs.

Shiatsu helps to keep open the communication between body, mind, emotion and spirit.

THE MAIN TECHNIQUES

PALMING

Palming is the simplest and most widely used technique in shiatsu. Palm pressure is gentle but firm, creating a supporting and soothing effect on any tense or vulnerable areas of the body.

Allow your hands to be relaxed so that your fingers can follow the contours of whatever part of the body you contact, then lean your body-weight through your palm, holding and waiting for the connection between your two palms. Lean back and without breaking contact, slide your hand along the body and lean forward again, creating stationary and perpendicular pressure.

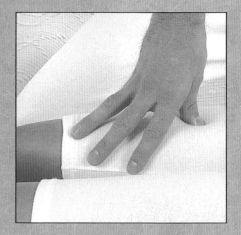

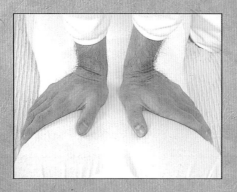

THUMBING

Thumb pressure is far more precise and penetrating than palming, and is used for working the points along the meridians. Place your thumbpads on the points. Use your extended fingers for support, so that the thumb remains straight. Lean your body forward so that most of the pressure is transferred through the thumbs. Make sure your nails are quite short to practise this technique or you may hurt your partner.

SIMPLE SHIATSU SESSION

The following sequences have been arranged so that each technique can flow smoothly into the next. Ideally the whole treatment should be experienced as a complete uninterrupted unit, not as a collection of separate movements. To achieve this, always maintain contact with your partner and make the transitions from one technique to the next with ease and fluency.

YANG

Position yourself at your partner's side. Take some time to centre yourself, clearing your mind so you can focus on your partner.

1 *Gently and firmly lay your hand on the small of your partner's back. This contact is an important time for both receiver and giver to attune to each other's energy. Use this time to assess the needs of your partner; feel the quality of the energy, physically, emotionally and spiritually. This can focus your intention in all the techniques to follow.*

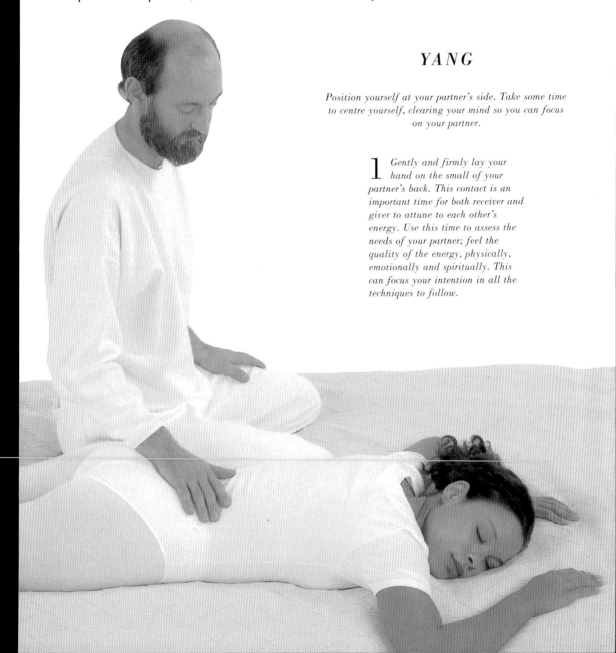

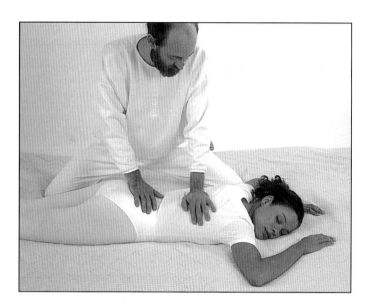

Left: This technique helps to disperse tension throughout, thus encouraging the energy to flow. It is useful to observe how your partner's body is moving. You will quickly be able to diagnose areas which may need more attention by simply observing which parts of the body are not moving as you rock.

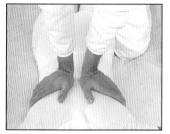

2 *Turn to face your partner and place the heel of the hands in the space between the shoulder blade and spine. With your knees apart begin to rock back and forth from your Hara (centre of the lower abdomen) and let the movement transfer through your hands so your partner's entire body moves in a*

wave-like motion. Continue to perform the rocking technique, working all the way down to the sacrum (lower back), moving the hands down the back in sequence.

Repeat two or three times and then repeat the same movements on the other side of the spine.

3 *Come up on to one knee, keeping an open posture. Placing your palms no higher than shoulder-blade level, on your receiver's "out" breath, bring your body-weight forward applying perpendicular pressure.*

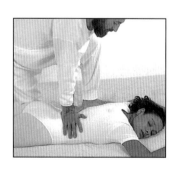

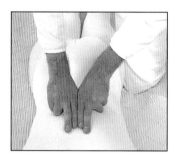

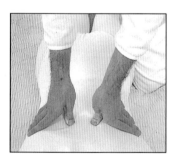

4 *Work down the back, moving a palm's width each time, and moving your body position to maintain perpendicular pressure. As you move below the ribs you may want to decrease the pressure slightly, as the internal organs are less protected here.*

5 *Having relaxed the back you can now locate the bladder meridian, which has a structural and energetic relationship with the nervous system. Measure two fingers' width from the centre of the spine and one hand's width down from the top of the shoulder.*

6 *Using the thumbs apply pressure at the points between the ribs. Thumb pressure is much more concentrated than palming. If you are unsure about how much pressure is appropriate, simply ask your partner how it feels.*

LEGS

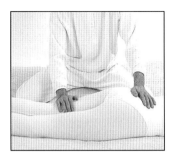

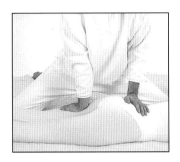

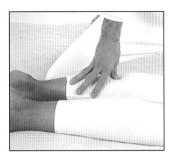

1 *Move your body down level to and facing your partner's legs. With your support hand on the lower back (sacrum), your messenger hand rocks and kneads simultaneously down the near-side thigh and calf several times.*

2 *Next palm down the leg, avoiding pressure on the backs of the knees.*

3 *Now thumb down the path of the bladder meridian. Depending on the length of the leg you may need to adjust your position. To avoid over-stretching, you can also move your support hand to just above the knee.*

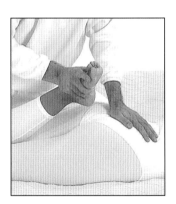

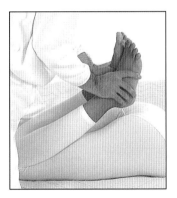

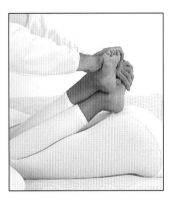

4 *With one hand on the sacrum, use the other hand to bring the foot gently back toward the buttocks, taking into consideration the leg's stretching capacity. Hold for a few seconds and then release.*

5 *Clasp both feet together and bend the legs, bringing the feet toward the buttocks. Hold this position for a few seconds and notice which foot goes closest to the buttocks to assess pelvic balance.*

6 *Cross this foot under the other foot and press them toward the buttocks on the "out" breath. Hold for several seconds then reverse the crossed legs and bend toward the buttocks once again.*

After these movements you will probably notice that the bending capacity of the legs has become more equal and the pelvis is more balanced.

Move round to the other side of the body and repeat the rocking, kneading, palming and thumbing on the other leg.

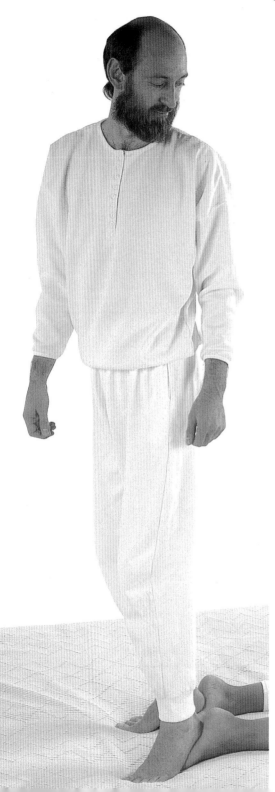

WORKING ON THE FEET

When "walking" on the feet make sure your position is well balanced as excess pressure or loss of balance may cause your partner pain.

Both the giving and receiving of pressure on the feet is very relaxing, and perfectly safe and easy to perform as long as you don't make any sudden or unexpected movements. Keep your body upright and relaxed as if you were going for a walk.

If there is too much of a gap between your partner's ankle and the floor, or the feet don't turn inward symmetrically, you may have to leave this technique out.

1 *Turn around so that your back is facing your partner and stand on both feet, shifting your weight from foot to foot. Control the movement from your hips.*

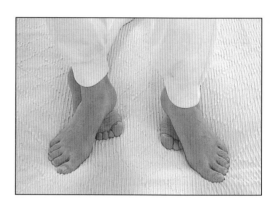

2 *Keep in one position and shift your weight back and forth from left to right several times and repeat on various areas of the feet.*

As with all the techniques, remember to observe your partner's facial expressions and breathing. These are obvious indications of how the receiver is feeling. Don't forget at any time that it's a human being you are working with, not just a body.

General pressure to the sole of the feet helps to stimulate the internal organs through the reflex areas and meridians. Walking on the feet is particularly good for grounding someone with too much mental activity.

YIN

Gently assist your partner to turn over into the supine position (on their back). Lying in this position we can be psychologically, emotionally and physically open, but we can also feel quite vulnerable. It is important to bear this in mind as you work to establish reassurance and trust.

Position yourself at your partner's side. Place one hand on your partner's waist, and the other hand on the abdomen with the heel of the hand just below the navel. Take a moment to listen with your hand to the rhythm of your partner's body. Feel the rise and fall of your partner's breath. Share the breath. This establishes a level of trust so

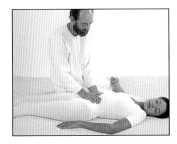

that you will be sensitive to any vulnerabilities or pains that might become manifest.

Gently palm around the abdomen in a clockwise direction. If you can coordinate your movements with your partner's "out" breath you should find that your partner gradually allows you to apply more pressure.

LEGS

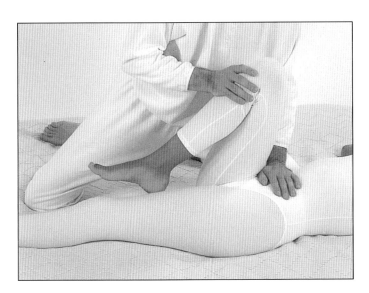

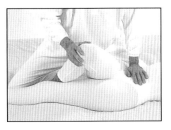

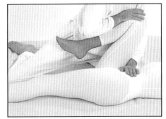

1 Change your position to face across your partner, placing your uppermost hand on the Hara (lower abdomen). Place your other hand on the inside of the knee allowing your fingers to curl under the joint. Leaning back, simply allow your body weight to lift the leg. There should be very little effort involved in this. As the leg comes up, slide your hand from the inside of the knee to the upper shin.

2,3 Rotate the leg out from the body, focusing on the hip joint. Start with small circular movements and, releasing the leg as much as possible, gradually increase the rotation to the fullest range.

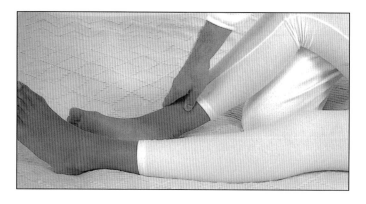

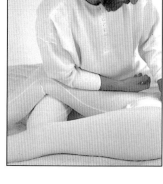

4 *Place the leg so that it rests comfortably with the toes at the level of the opposite ankle, with the spleen meridian uppermost. You may prop it up either with* your leg underneath or a cushion. Palm up the inside of the calf along the Yin meridians to the knee. Thumb up the calf from the ankle to the knee.

5 *Use your forearm to continue the pressure up the thigh. Rotate the leg once again then move down to your partner's feet.*

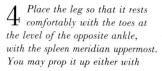

=== **CAUTION** ===

Do not give shiatsu on the spleen meridian during pregnancy if miscarriage is likely. Do not work below the knees in any pregnancy.

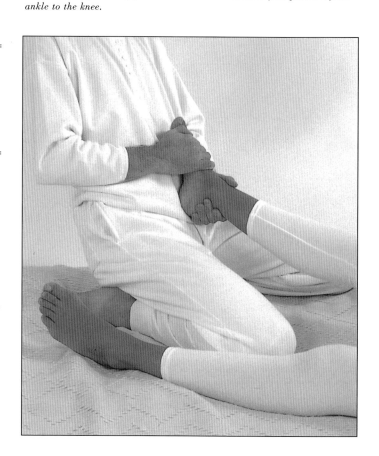

6 *Cup underneath the ankle in one hand. Place the other hand on top of the ankle. Bring your Hara into contact with the sole of the foot. Grasp it firmly and rotate your body from the hips. As you move your partner's body will move with yours.*

Repeat all the techniques on the opposite leg and complete this section of the sequence with your hand back on your receiver's Hara.

SHOULDERS, ARMS AND HANDS

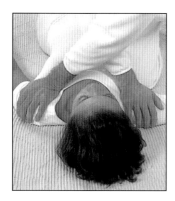

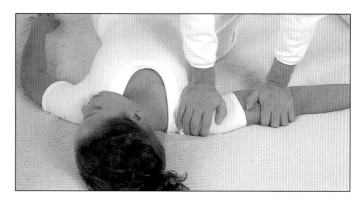

1 *Kneeling up, bring your free hand to your partner's furthest shoulder. Place your other hand on the near shoulder. Your arms should now be crossed. With your receiver's "out" breath, lean forward on your hands, opening up the shoulder and chest area.*

2 *Maintain the support of the shoulder nearest you. With the other hand, as in the treatment of the legs, begin by gently rocking and kneading the arms from the shoulder to the hand. Position the arm at right angles to the body*

with the palms facing up. Then palm down the arm, avoiding pressure on the elbow joint. Follow by thumbing down the middle of the arm to the palm along the heart protector meridian.

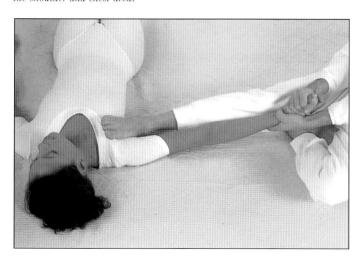

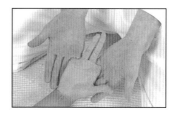

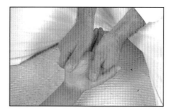

3 *Grasp the wrist and move your body so that your outstretched leg is parallel to the arm, your foot resting comfortably against the*

upper torso. Gently lean back stretching the arm, giving counterpressure with your foot.

4,5 *Link your little fingers inside your partner's index and little finger to stretch open the palm. Your thumbs are then naturally placed to work into the palm with circular movements.*

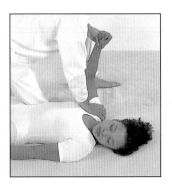

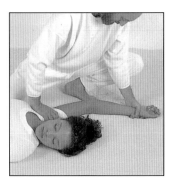

6 Place the support hand on the shoulder, tucking your thumb into the armpit. Hold the wrist, lift and loosen the shoulder joint.

7 Step forward with your outside leg, stretching your partner's arm to the floor above the head.

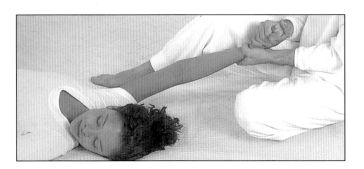

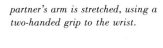

8 Move your body so that by gently leaning back your

partner's arm is stretched, using a two-handed grip to the wrist.

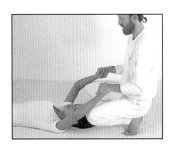

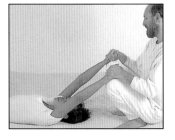

9 Pick up your partner's other hand and rest the forearms on your knees.

10 Lean back, allowing your knees to slide up the forearms to the wrists. On the "out" breath, this makes a powerful stretch for the shoulders and chest.

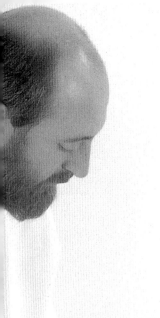

Repeat all the techniques on the opposite arm: stretching, rocking, kneading, palming, thumbing and massaging the hands.

To finish return again to the Hara (lower abdomen area). Simply holding for a minute or two gives your partner time to feel the changes that have occurred.

Break this final contact very slowly and if appropriate cover your partner with a blanket. Give your partner some time to experience how he or she feels.

One of the great benefits of shiatsu is that it encourages self-awareness. It is often in the still moments of a session, when we are just being with our partner, that both giver and receiver can have the most profound insights.

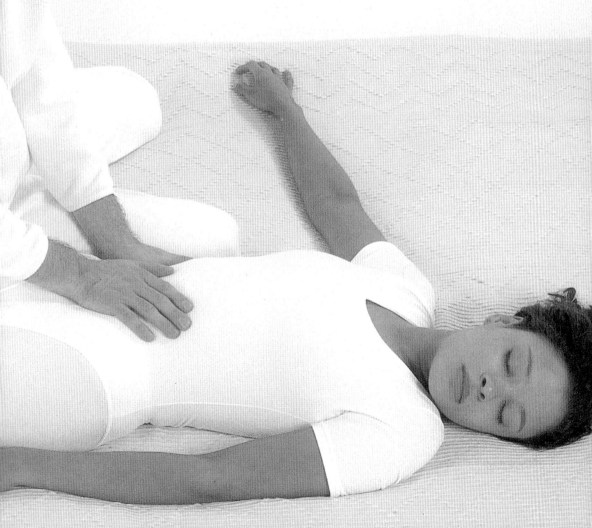

USEFUL ADDRESSES

AROMATHERAPY

ORGANIZATIONS

These organizations will provide information about accredited therapists and courses. Please always send a stamped, self-addressed envelope when writing.

Aromatherapy Organizations Council
3 Latymer Close
Braybrooke
Market Harborough
Leicester LE16 8LN
Tel: 0455 615466

Holistic Aromatherapy Foundation
16 Sunnyhill Road
London SW16 2VH
Tel: 081 664 6150

International Federation of Aromatherapists
Department of Continuing Education
The Royal Masonic Hospital
Ravenscourt Park
London W6 0TN
Tel: 081 846 8066

International Society of Professional Aromatherapists
41 Leicester Road
Hinckley
Leicestershire LE10 1LW
Tel: 0455 637987

National Holistic Aromatherapy Association
PO Box 18622
Boulder
CO 803-0622
USA
Tel: (303) 258 2791

International Federation of Aromatherapists
197 7th Street
Midland
Ontario L4R 3Z4
Canada

Australian Natural Therapists Association
PO Box 522
Sutherland
NSW 2232
Australia

Institute of Clinical Aromatherapy
PO Box 734
Skellenbosch 7599
South Africa

MAIL ORDER SUPPLIERS

Nina Ashby Aromatherapy
29 Arundel Road
Croydon CR0 2ER
Tel: 081 689 3949

Culpeper Ltd
Hadstock Road
Linton
Cambridge CB1 6NJ
Tel: 0223 894054

Kobashi
50 High Street
Ide
Devon EX2 9RW
Tel: 0392 217628

Eve Taylor
22 Bromley Road
London SE6 2TP
Tel: 081 690 2149

The Body Shop
Watersmead Business Park
Littlehampton
West Sussex BN17 6LS
Tel: 0903 731500

Neal's Yard Remedies
15 Neal's Yard
London WC2H 9DP
Tel: 071 379 0141

Rachel Stewart
Avalon Aromatics
20 Springfield Road
London SW19 7AL
Tel: 081 947 1567

The Body Shop (USA)
45 Holsehill Road
Cedar Knolls
NJ 07927
USA
Tel: 1 800 541 2535

Quintessence Aromatherapy
PO Box 4996
Boulder
CO 80306
USA

Just Good Scents
206 Collingwood Court
Edmurton
Alberta T5T 0H5
Canada

Essentially Yours
Factory 35
65-7 Canterbury Road
Montrose 3765
Victoria
Australia

RESIDENTIAL TREATMENTS

Henlow Grange
Henlow
Bedfordshire SG16 6DB
Tel: 0426 811111

Grayshott Hall
Headley Road
Grayshott
Nr. Hindhead
Surrey GU26 6JJ
Tel: 0428 604331

Champneys
Wiggington
Tring
Hertfordshire HP23 6HY
Tel: 0442 873155

**HAIR AND BEAUTY
THERAPY TREATMENTS**

**Michaeljohn/
The Ragdale Clinic**
25 Albermarle Street
London W1X 3FA
Tel: 071 629 6969

Michaeljohn
14 North
414 North Camden Drive
Beverly Hills
CA 90210
USA
Tel: 310 278 8333

SHIATSU

**The British School of
Shiatsu-Do**
188 Old Street
London EC1V 9FR
Tel: 071 251 0831

The Shiatsu Society
14 Oakdene Road
Redhill
Surrey RH1 6BT
Tel: 0737 767896

Clive Ives
45 Broderick Road
London SW17 7DX
Tel: 081 672 0477

**The American Shiatsu
Society**
44 Pear Street
Cambridge
MA 02139
USA

FURTHER READING

AROMATHERAPY

Micheline Arcier, *Aromatherapy*, Hamlyn, 1990

Patricia Davies, *Aromatherapy: An A-Z*, C. W. Daniel, 1988

Judith Jackson, *Aromatherapy*, Henry Holt and Co, 1986

Marguerite Maury, *Guide to Aromatherapy: The Secret of Life and Youth*, C. W. Daniel, 1989

Shirley Price, *Practical Aromatherapy*, Thorsons, 1987
Aromatherapy for Common Ailments, Gaia Books, 1991

Maggie Tisserand, *Aromatherapy for Women*, Thorsons, 1989

Robert Tisserand, *The Art of Aromatherapy*, C. W. Daniel 1977
Aromatherapy for Everyone, Penguin, 1990

SHIATSU

Saul Goodman, *The Shiatsu Practitioner's Manual*, Infitech Publications, 1986

Shizuto Masunaga, *Zen Shiatsu*, Japan Publications, 1977

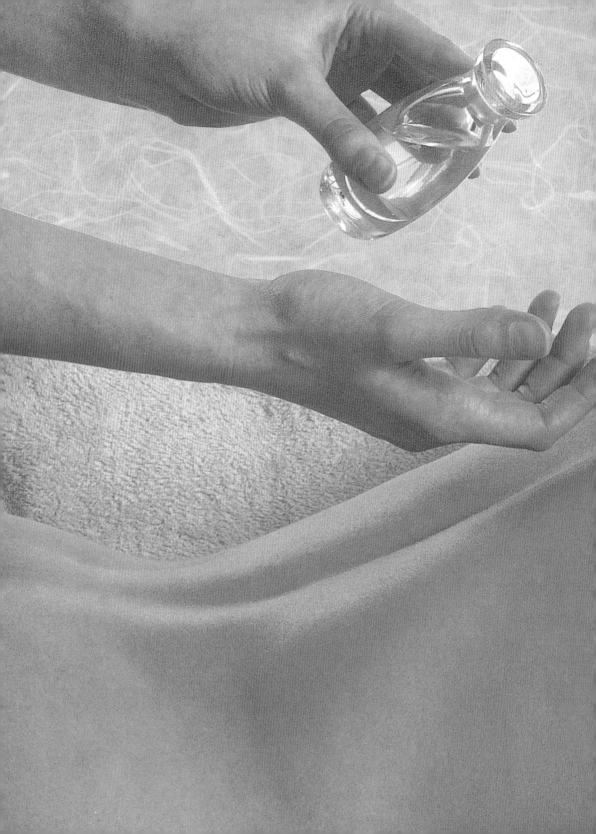

MASSAGE

≈

Everyone enjoys massage. From
babies to the elderly, from sportsmen
and women to friends and lovers, all
can benefit from this powerful form of
communication. An effective aid to
relaxation, massage helps to smoothe
away stress, unknotting tense and
aching muscles, relieving headaches
and helping sleep problems. But
massage is also invigorating: it
improves the functioning of many of
the body's systems, promotes healing
and tones muscles, leaving you with a
feeling of renewed energy. By
mastering a few simple techniques and
sequences, you will learn the language
of touch – a valuable gift for yourself
and others.

THE HUMAN TOUCH

The sense of touch is a powerful and highly sensitive form of communication. It is a natural reaction to reach out and touch, whether to feel the shape or texture of something, or to respond to another person, perhaps by comforting them. A mother cuddles her baby, family pets are stroked, sexual partners caress, and if we accidentally knock a limb we instinctively "rub it better".

To touch someone can mean various things in different cultures. There are many social restraints which inhibit touching in public. For us, a formal handshake, nod of the head, and even a peck on each cheek are all recognized forms of greeting, and yet you can carry them out without showing any real emotion. Indeed, our rather formal approach to physical contact is contrary to our most basic instincts and needs. Fortunately, we are now rediscovering the healing power of massage and other touch therapies which have been understood in other cultures for thousands of years.

THE DEVELOPMENT OF MASSAGE

History shows that although the early Egyptians made references to the benefits of massage, the Chinese were among the first to recognize its healing value at around 3000 BC. Roman and Greek philosophers and physicians prescribed it both for its restorative powers after battle and for general preservation of the body and mind. Although the Romans believed in its curative powers, the art of massage also became part of a daily ritual for relaxation. After bathing, oils would be used to anoint the body from head to toe, followed by a luxurious massage.

Herbalists throughout history have used massage to heal body and soul, both by applying balms and by laying their own hands on the afflicted to expel evil spirits and clear the mind. It wasn't until the eighteenth and nineteenth centuries, though, that massage became popular throughout Europe, thanks to the work of Per Henrik Ling (1776–1839). Ling was a Swede who travelled to China and returned with a detailed insight into their massage techniques. From these he developed his own system of massage based on a variety of movements, involving pressure, friction, vibration and rotation.

This wealth of practical knowledge soon spread, and medical and non-medical professions worldwide began exploring the benefits of massage. This eventually established the basis of massage today, which in many ways remains much the same now as those early Swedish techniques.

Along with basic massage we are now experiencing a

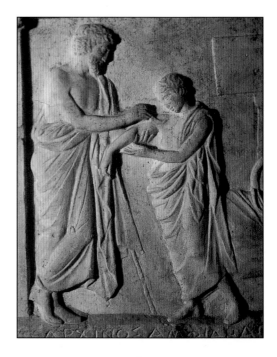

revival of interest in many of the ancient arts which place such great importance on touch. These include aromatherapy, reflexology and shiatsu – all distinctive natural therapies which have a specific role to play in "alternative" health-care.

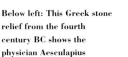

Below left: This Greek stone relief from the fourth century BC shows the physician Aesculapius treating a patient by "rubbing", as recommended by Hippocrates.

Right: As Europe emerged from the Middle Ages, massage once again became part of the bathing ritual, as shown in this sixteenth-century German woodcut of a public bath house.

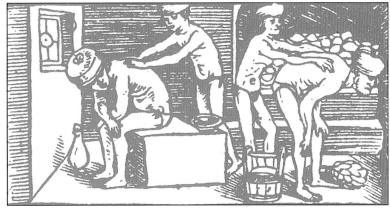

EFFECTS OF MASSAGE

Massage can stimulate and relax the body and the mind. The skin, blood and lymphatic systems are stimulated, which boosts circulation, aids cellular renewal and removes toxic wastes. As tense muscles relax, stiff joints loosen and nerves are soothed, an all-over feeling of relaxation and well-being comes about.

The Nervous System

The nervous system is a highly complex network which relays messages from the brain to the rest of the body. The part of the nervous system which regulates many physiological functions leaves the brain at the base of the skull and runs down the spinal cord, protected by the spine's bony vertebrae. Millions of nerve endings run throughout the body, controlling much of the way it functions. Depending on the depth of the massage movements used, the nerve endings can be stimulated or soothed.

The Skin

With massage comes an increase in blood circulation. This helps the exfoliation of superficial dead skin cells, tones the skin and encourages its renewal process. Massage helps maintain the collagen fibres, which give skin its elasticity and strength, and keep wrinkles at bay. The activity of the sweat and sebaceous glands, which lubricate and moisturize the skin, is regulated.

Muscles

With the increase in blood flow, the blood's vital nutrients circulate more efficiently. Massage is popular with sportsmen and women because it can improve muscle tone, restore mobility, and ensure the elimination of waste products after exercise. With regular massage, strains and sprains heal more rapidly, while calf cramps and stiff muscles can become a thing of the past. Massage before an exercise session will help loosen and warm up the muscles, or afterwards it will ease sore, aching limbs.

Circulation and Lymphatic Systems

By dilating the blood vessels, massage increases the blood circulation. A good circulatory system means that an efficient supply of the blood's constituents, including oxygen and nutrients, reaches the billions of individual cells. This is vital for the healthy functioning of the whole body, from the muscles to internal organs such as the kidneys and liver.

At the same time the increase in blood circulation helps accelerate the lymphatic system, which absorbs and eliminates waste substances. Unlike the blood circulation, which has the heart to pump it round, the lymphatic system has no pump of its own and is dependent on muscular action for its efficiency. Massage is an important means of speeding up the flow of the lymph, encouraging a more effective filtering and elimination of waste throughout the body. An efficient lymphatic system provides the body with a strong immune system to fight against infections and disease.

Digestion

Massage mobilizes the digestive system so that the processes of assimilation and elimination are improved, helping problems like constipation and flatulence. The digestive system is quick to respond to stress, and the reduction in anxiety and tension which comes with regular massage has a regulating effect on the digestion.

THE BASIC TECHNIQUES

When many people think of massage they picture the vigorous pummelling and slapping often associated with puritanical health spas. In truth, firm massage can be highly beneficial without causing discomfort. Alternate firm and gentle flowing strokes to create a combination that will alleviate tension and muscular aches and pains whilst energizing and invigorating the body.

In Swedish massage there are four basic types of movement. Familiarize yourself with these different techniques before beginning the step-by-step, whole-body massage.

EFFLEURAGE

Effleurage describes long, soothing, stroking movements using the flat of the hand (or fingers if working on small areas). These are often used to apply oil evenly to the body. You can use one hand on its own or with the other providing support on top of it, both hands simultaneously, or one hand alternating with the other.

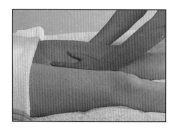

Relax the hands and mould them to the contours of the body. Apply slightly more pressure when you take the stroke in the direction of the heart to improve circulation and lymph flow. If you are working away from the heart, keep the pressure firmer on the return stroke. The movements should be fairly slow and continuous. Keep the hands in contact with your partner between strokes.

Effleurage is used to start off a massage, soothing the nerve endings and helping your partner get used to your touch. It is used again at the end of a massage for a relaxing finish. In between, *effleurage* movements provide an important link between other more stimulating strokes and are used to make first contact with a new area of the body. If you feel hesitant about what to do next, you can always insert some *effleurage*, so the continuity is not lost.

You repeat *effleurage* strokes several times. Each time try to start the first complete stroke with fairly light pressure, then apply slightly more pressure with the next complete stroke. Where there are larger muscle areas, such as the thighs and back, you can apply the most pressure for a more stimulating effect.

PETRISSAGE

Petrissage describes a number of movements which involve various ways of kneading, rolling and picking up the skin and muscles. These firm and strengthen the structures by stimulating the deep layers of tissue, and increasing the supply of blood to the area. They also improve the flow of lymph.

Generally a single group of muscles, or an individual muscle, is worked on at one time. The basic kneading action is very similar to kneading dough.

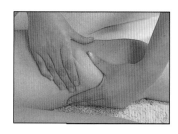

For *petrissage*, start with your fingers pointing away from you, press down with the palm, grasp the flesh between fingers and thumb and push it toward the other hand. As you release the first hand your second hand grasps the flesh and pushes it back toward the first hand. It is a continuous action, alternating the hands to squeeze and release.

With light kneading you are tackling the top muscle layers, whilst firmer kneading works on the deeper muscles, easing taut muscles and breaking down congested tissues to help the elimination of waste products.

FRICTION

Friction, or "connective tissue massage", is a penetrating circular movement which applies deep direct pressure to one particular site of muscular tension, using the thumb, fingertips or knuckles. It is a valuable technique for concentrating on specific areas of tightness and muscle spasm in the back.

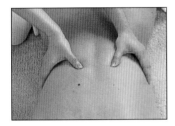

As you make the circular rotations you should actually feel the underlying tissues moving; you are not simply sliding over the skin's surface.

A variation on circular friction pressures is static pressure, where you lean gradually into the muscle, slowly deepening the pressure without the rotation action. Press for a few seconds, then gradually release.

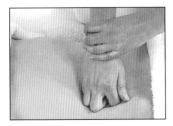

Another friction movement is knuckling: use the knuckles in a loosely clenched fist to produce rippling, circular motions. This is used to release tension up the sides of the spine and in other areas. Remember not to work right on top of the spine bone.

TAPOTEMENT

Tapotement, or percussion movements, are fast and stimulating. They include cupping, hacking, pounding (also called pummelling), which all sound like painful practices but when carried out properly should certainly not cause bruising or pain. (Don't use *tapotement* on particularly bony areas or on broken or varicose veins.) For all the movements, remember to keep the hands and wrists relaxed. All the percussion techniques are fast, precision actions, bringing one hand quickly after the other into contact with your partner. It is particularly important at the beginning to ask your partner whether you are applying the right degree of pressure.

These sequences stimulate the blood circulation, tone and help strengthen sagging skin and muscles. In particular *tapotement* can tighten up soft tissue areas, such as thighs and buttocks, which are prone to cellulite.

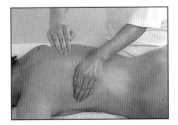

For cupping, gently curve the hands to make a loose cupped shape, bending at the knuckles while keeping the fingers straight and firm. Do not bend the fingers too far over. Using the cupped palm, make a bouncy, brisk, cupping action against a fleshy area, alternating the hands quickly. The fast, cupping action creates a suction against the skin. Try this movement on the back, buttocks and thighs.

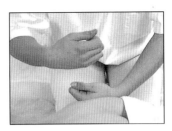

For pounding (or pummelling), loosely clench your fists, but keep the wrists relaxed. You can use the wrists in two ways: either striking your partner with the outer edges of the loose fist or with the front of the knuckles. Either way, the speed and rhythm of the movement is similar: brisk and firm, alternating the hands, without thumping your partner too enthusiastically. Once again, keep to the fleshier parts of the body, particularly cellulite zones such as hips, buttocks and thighs.

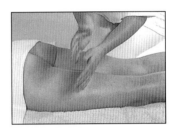

In hacking, the outer edge of the hand is used to stimulate the area by striking it quickly with alternate hands. You need to practise a brisk, bouncing movement, working rhythmically and rapidly over a fleshy area of the body. You need to have very relaxed wrists and fingers, and use the sides of the palm rather than the fingers. Used over the buttocks and thighs, hacking tones up muscles and disperses fluid.

Intersperse these brisk movements with the gentler, *effleurage* strokes, then go back to the pounding or pummelling for as long as you both feel comfortable.

WHOLE-BODY MASSAGE

Our whole-body massage is a comprehensive, top-to-toe sequence based on Swedish massage techniques, specially adapted for home practice. As a beginner you may find the full sequence too tiring at first. Until your hands and wrists build up their strength and you get used to positioning your own body comfortably to perform the massage, it is best to work on just a few parts of the body, such as the back of the legs, back and shoulders, or to perform fewer movements on each part of the body. Your partner will find it more relaxing if you perform one or two types of movement thoroughly rather than keep changing the strokes after a few seconds to cover all the steps. Always include *effleurage* strokes to begin and end a sequence, and never leave the body unbalanced – if you work on one leg or arm, you should repeat the same movements on the other side of the body.

COMFORT AND CLOTHING

If you are going to massage on the floor, put down a thick layer of blankets or towels, or a futon, to provide your partner with a firm, comfortable cushion. There is nothing more likely to reverse the relaxation process than a hard surface, a cold room and noise. Choose a quiet time, when you won't be disturbed. Your partner may need the room quite a lot warmer than you might expect. Being massaged on the floor might be extremely comfortable for your partner, but it can put a strain on the masseur's back and knees so, if you prefer, set up the same cushioning surface on a large table. It is not a good idea to massage on a bed – the give of a soft mattress can counteract much of your effort.

Have ready several towels, so that you can cover areas of the body which are not being worked on. Often a sense of modesty is crucial to relaxation, and the towels will also keep your partner warm. Move the towels around to cover most of the body, and especially an area you have just

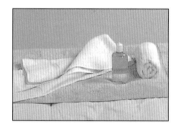

finished working on. You will need a cushion or towel to support the head, and it can be helpful to put a roll of towel under the knees when your partner is lying on their back. This relaxes the lower back. When your partner turns over on to the front, a towel under the chest can improve comfort.

Massage in loose-fitting clothes, with soft-soled, flat shoes, or work in bare feet. Take off rings and jewellery, so there is nothing to distract your partner, and make sure your nails are short! The more relaxed you are, as the masseur, the better. If you feel keyed up, try some deep, regular breathing exercises before you start. Take a few stretches, shake your hands to loosen any tension, and you're ready to start.

OILS

There are several oils which are appropriate for body massage. Stick to vegetable oils, rather than mineral oils such as baby oil. Grapeseed, sunflower or almond oil are good, basic vegetable oils, which are light and therefore not too sticky. Jojoba is a good oil for the face, especially if your partner has oily skin. Avoid oils with strong smells, such as olive oil. Also try experimenting by adding a little avocado, apricot' or peach kernel oil if you wish, or buy ready-mixed massage oil.

Measure 3–4 tablespoons (45–60 ml) oil into a saucer or small container before starting your massage. You will quickly get used to how much oil to apply. The amount varies with the dryness of the skin, and how readily it absorbs the oil, but in general you need enough to facilitate the strokes without applying so much that your hands simply slide over the skin. If you need to apply more oil during a sequence, simply smooth a little oil into the palms of your hands and do some extra *effleurage* strokes.

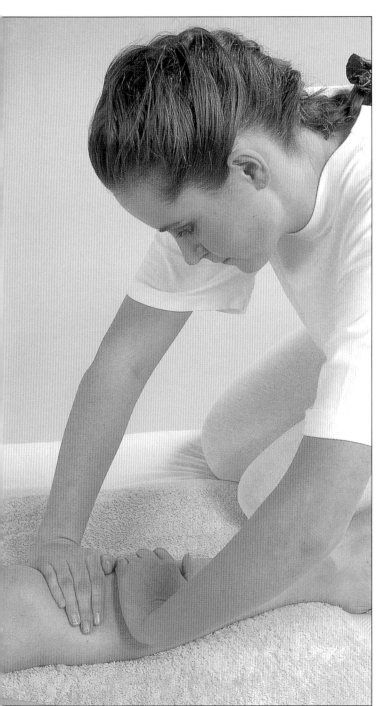

Exchanging a regular basic massage is a luxury for both giver and receiver. However, specific problems should be tackled by a trained practitioner. Never massage right on top of the spine. Working down each side of the bony spinal column is fine, and produces many benefits, but you should avoid working directly on top of the spine.

There are occasions when it is not appropriate to massage. Avoid if there are any of the following conditions:

● heart condition
● high blood pressure
● bacterial or viral infection
● nausea or abdominal pain
● severe back pain which may be caused by the spine, especially if there are shooting pains in other limbs
● temperature or fever
● open wound or skin infection
● cancer
● post-operative recovery

If you are in any doubt, it is always best to check with your doctor first.

THE FULL MASSAGE SEQUENCE

Front of Body:
1 Legs 2 Feet and ankles
3 Arms and hands 4 Chest, shoulders and neck 5 Face
6 Abdomen and waist
Back of Body:
7 Legs and buttocks
8 Back and shoulders

FRONT OF BODY

*The full massage begins with the front of the body, so your partner should
lie face up with cushions or rolled towels wherever needed for support.*

LEGS

Since legs carry the full body weight, the bones and
muscles in the legs are the largest and strongest we
have. A good leg massage can not only help to relieve
strain and tension in the legs, but can benefit the well-
being of the whole body. It's not unknown for backache
to be traced to problems in the legs, and for a good leg
massage to help alleviate the pain.

Leg massage stimulates both the blood circulation
and the lymphatic system, and done regularly it helps to
prevent varicose veins. Any congestion in the lower legs
will be lessened with effleurage movements taken up
toward the lymph nodes at the back of the knee and in
the groin. If legs feel puffy or swollen to the touch,
make sure you use the gentlest of pressure. Firm
massage on the larger muscles, such as those round the
thighs, can dispel tiredness and stimulate a sluggish
lymphatic system. Work more lightly over bony areas
such as the shins and knees.

VARICOSE VEINS

You need to take certain precautions
if your partner has varicose veins.
Never knead or put any pressure on
varicose veins, and only massage the
part of the leg which is higher than
the area with veins (that is, only
massage closer to the heart); never on
or below the vein.

EFFLEURAGE

1 *Below: Kneel beside your
partner's left ankle. With a
little oil in the palm of your hands,
start with your hands crossed over
the ankle, in readiness to begin
several long effleurage strokes. You
will need more oil if the legs are
particularly hairy or dry, but don't
add too much in the first instance.*

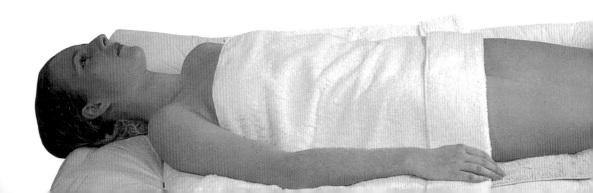

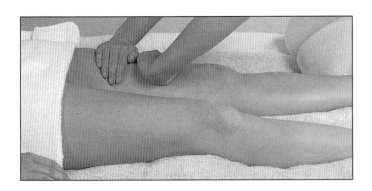

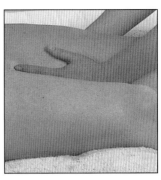

2 *Keeping your hands crossed over the leg, slide the palms up the front of the leg, over the knee* and up to the thigh, in one continuous, sweeping movement to oil the front of the leg evenly.

3 *Turn the hands outward round the hip, separate them and bring the hands back down each side of the thigh.*

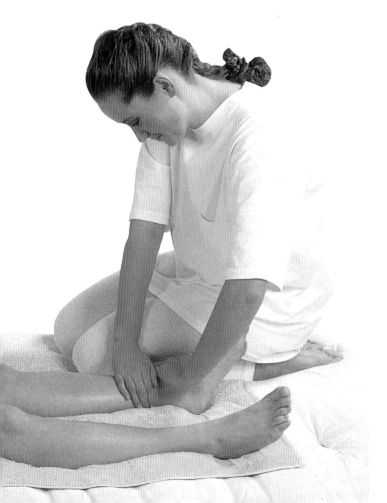

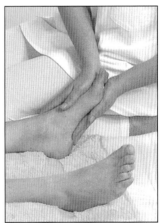

4 *Continue to sweep the hands back to the ankle, and then over the foot to the toes. Then place your hands crossed over the ankle again, ready to repeat the entire movement.*

Use some more oil if necessary, and this time use slightly firmer pressure on the upward stroke, then lighter again for the return. The stroke is smooth and continuous throughout.

Repeat the sequence over the whole leg once again.

THIGHS

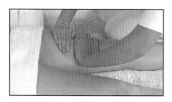

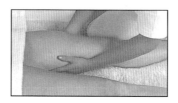

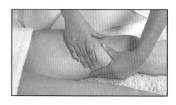

1 Bring both hands up to just above the knee and move them up together, pressing the muscles firmly toward the upper thigh. You should be applying enough pressure to see movement in the muscles.

2 At the top of the thigh separate the hands and using lighter pressure come down either side of the leg to the knee.

3 Begin kneading the inner thigh with both hands. Squeeze, then release the muscles, picking up and rolling them as you do so. Continue the kneading action over the top and outside thigh.

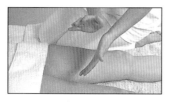

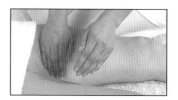

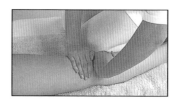

4 Now use a hacking movement all over the thigh. Briskly strike the area with the outside edge of one hand after another, using short, sharp movements. Keep a fast repetition going.

5 Continue with cupping all over the thigh, working quickly. Expect quite a loud cupping sound, but check with your partner that the strokes are not too powerful.

6 Begin at the knee and do some effleurage strokes up to the top of the thigh, sweeping the hands outward and back down to the knee, to soothe the area after the series of stimulating movements.

KNEES

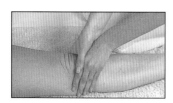

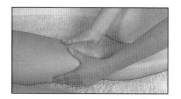

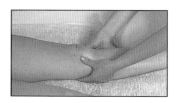

1 Place both hands just below the knee. Lightly massage round the kneecap, using your fingertips to work gently into the muscles. Repeat three times.

2 Starting with your thumbs above the kneecap, with your hands under the knee for support, slowly draw them lightly round the outside of the kneecap and release. Repeat this movement three times.

3 Support the back of the knee with your hands and use your thumbs to circle gently round the kneecap, working downward. Return to the top of the knee and repeat three times.

4 *Right: Raise the height of your hands above the knee. Work round the kneecap with one hand, loosening the muscles with your thumb and fingers. Use gentle, circular rotations to cover the area thoroughly.*

You may find it easier to support your wrist with the other hand.

Do some more effleurage strokes, sweeping them up from the ankle to just below the kneecap and back down to the ankle. Repeat this several times.

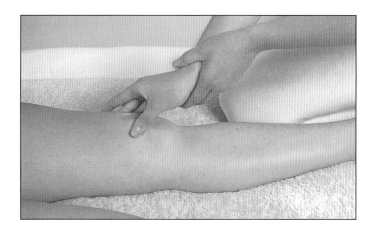

CALVES

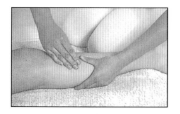

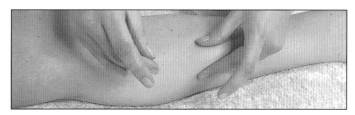

1 *Knead the calf muscles. Squeeze and release them, working from the ankle up to the knee.*

2 *Lightly and quickly pinch the fleshy part of the calf with the fingers and thumbs, one hand after the other. Check with your* partner that you are not pinching too hard, although this needs to be felt to be effective.

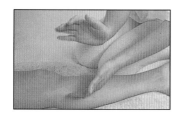

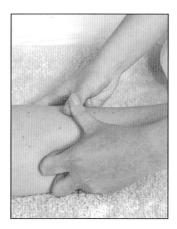

4 *Left: Starting at the ankle and crossing your thumbs on top of the shin for support, with loose knuckles make semi-circular kneading movements, working up and down the calf.*

Finish the leg with some effleurage movements from ankle to thigh.

3 *Using the outside edge of both hands, alternately and rhythmically strike the calf muscles, working up and down the entire length, but keeping away from the bony shin area itself. Keep the hacking action short and brisk.*

FEET AND ANKLES

A foot massage is particularly relaxing after the legs have been worked on. It can alleviate anxiety and stress, stimulate the circulation and nervous system, help insomniacs to sleep, and energize anyone feeling tired and lethargic. There are thousands of nerve endings in the foot, particularly on the sole. Try to include the ankles too, to improve their flexibility.

Change the pressure of the strokes to suit your partner, remembering that deeper pressure tends to revitalize whereas gentle strokes increase relaxation throughout the entire person. When working on the feet it is best to use only a very little oil, otherwise your hands will slide around and tickle. If your partner's feet are hot and sticky, use a little talcum powder instead.

Before starting, you may wish to raise your partner's knee slightly with a
rolled towel under them, to relax the muscles around the knee and
in the lower back.

FEET AND ANKLES

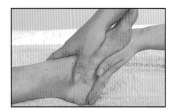

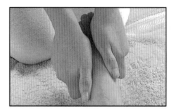

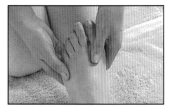

1 Kneel at your partner's feet. Starting with the hands at the ankle, gently slide your hands toward the tips of the toes and then release them. Repeat several times. If you are using oil, apply it with this stroke.

2 With the heels of your hand, give a good stretch to the top of the foot. Draw the heel toward the sides of the foot to give the stretch. Repeat a few times, working slightly further down the foot too.

3 Supporting the foot in both hands, find the furrow between each tendon and, using small, circular movements, work both thumbs up the tendons toward the ankle. Repeat three times on each tendon.

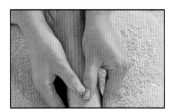

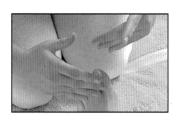

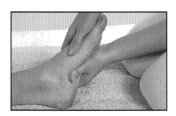

4 Resting the thumbs across the top of the ankle, work the fingers right round the ankle bone using light, circular movements.

5 Lightly tap the toes with your fingers to build up some gentle friction.

6 Now knead the foot firmly, working particularly well into the arch. You will need to use different parts of the hand, such as the heel, knuckle and thumbs.

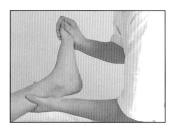

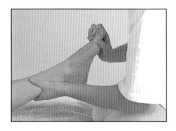

7,8 *Supporting the lower leg with your left hand, gently rotate the ankle three times in each direction, without forcing.*

9 *Right: Give the foot a gentle stretch backward and forward, to relax and flex the tendons. Supporting the back of the lower leg, use your other hand at the toes to push the foot gently away from you. To reverse the stretch take the hand over the top of the foot, and press the foot down, still supporting the lower leg with the other hand.*

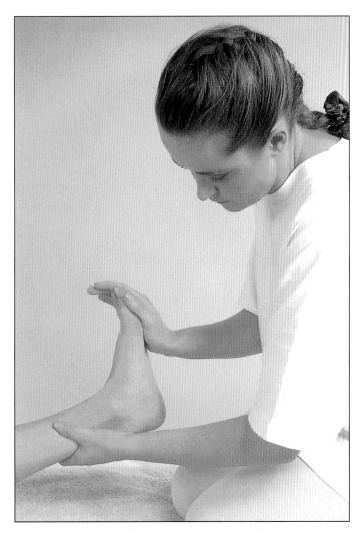

10 *Finish the foot and ankle sequence with some long sweeping, effleurage strokes from the top of the foot up the lower leg and back down to the foot, to help reintegrate the foot and the leg. Repeat several times, varying the pressure.*

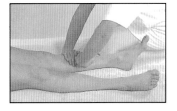

Move round your partner to kneel on the other side.
Repeat the entire sequence on the front of the other leg and the other foot.

ARMS AND HANDS

Arms and hands can hide the most powerful emotions. Tight, clenched arms and hands often reflect insecurity, self-protection and unresolved anger. Whether the posture is intentional or sub-conscious, tension in the arms can cause headaches, neck pain, and aching shoulders. Don't be put off if your partner's arms are slim and bony, there are still important muscle areas there.

A hand massage feels surprisingly good, almost on a par with having the feet massaged. A lot of tension creeps into the hands: a massage is a reminder of how it feels to relax them. Massaging the arms and hands can liberate and relax not only the muscles but also the pent-up emotions, as your partner starts to feel the wonderful sensation of letting go.

ARMS

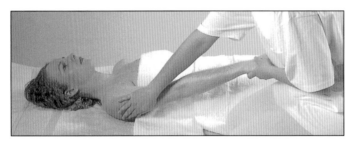
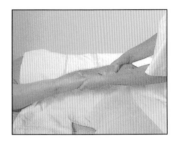

1 *Kneel halfway along your partner's right side. Holding the wrist with your left hand, lightly oil the arm using* effleurage *strokes, starting from the wrist and sweeping your hand up round the shoulder and down again. Repeat three times.*

2 *Changing hands, so that your partner's wrist is supported in your right hand, use the left hand to stroke gently from the wrist to the shoulder, and back down again. Repeat several times.*

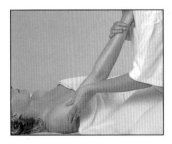
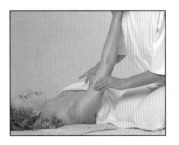
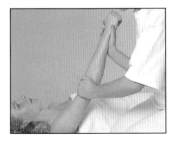

3 *Lift the arm and rest the hand on your right shoulder ready to start kneading. Support your partner's wrist with your left hand and use your right to knead lightly the muscles of the upper arm, working from elbow to shoulder.*

4 *Keeping your partner's hand supported by your shoulder, use the fingers of both hands to continue the kneading.*

5 *Still holding the arm across the front of your chest with your right hand, do some effleurage strokes from the elbow up to the shoulder and back down again. Repeat three times.*

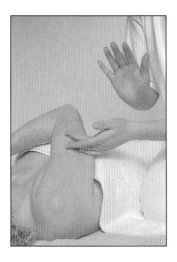

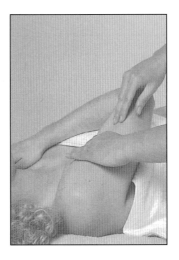

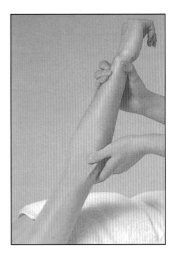

6 *Bend your partner's arm and rest the right hand on the left shoulder. Using the outside edge of your hands, do some short, brisk hacking on the outer and under sides of the arm.*

7 *With your partner's arm still bent, firmly knead the muscles of the upper arm with your right hand, using the left hand to keep your partner's arm stable.*

8 *Holding the wrist for support with your right hand, work round the outside of the elbow with your fingers and thumb, using smooth circular movements and covering the area thoroughly. As the elbows can get particularly dry you may need some more oil.*

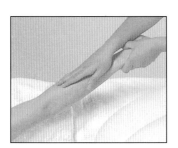

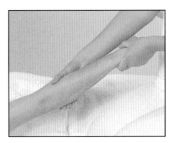

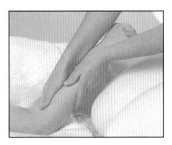

9 *To encourage further relaxation, hold the wrist with the left hand and do some effleurage strokes up and down the top of the forearm. Keep the pressure fairly firm.*

10 *Repeat these effleurage strokes on the inside of the forearm.*

11 *Rest your partner's elbow back on the towel. Supporting the weight of the lower arm in your left hand, use your right hand to knead the inside of the forearm, starting from the wrist. When you reach the elbow glide gently back to the wrist to begin again. Repeat three times.*

Finish the arm with a few effleurage strokes and then massage the hand and wrist (see the following pages) before moving on to the other arm.

HANDS AND WRISTS

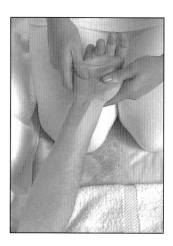

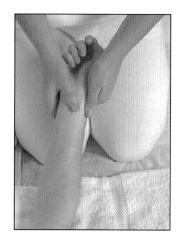

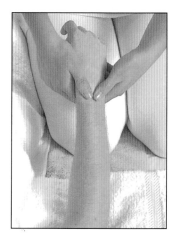

1 *Support your partner's hand in both hands and gently use the thumbs to knead the palm. This should be a continuous, circular action, with the thumbs alternately applying the pressure.*

2 *Rest your hands under your partner's wrist and use the thumbs to stroke outward round the wrist. Then work with the thumbs up the inner forearm toward the elbow, using circular movements.*

3 *Turn the hand over, supporting the wrist. Massage gently over the back of the wrist with your thumbs.*

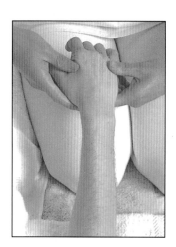

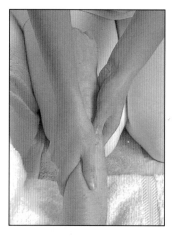

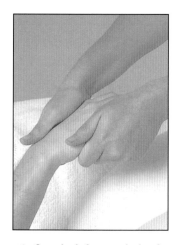

4 *Stroke up in between the tendons on the back of the hand with your thumbs, from knuckles to wrist, using light small circles. Repeat twice between each tendon.*

5 *Sweep the hands alternately up from the wrist toward the elbow, applying a fairly firm pressure with the inside edge of the hands. Repeat several times.*

6 *Come back down to the hand and stretch the back of the hand, drawing your hands out toward the sides.*

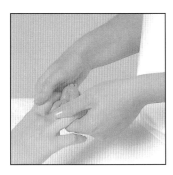
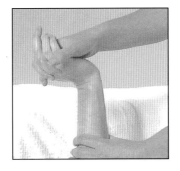
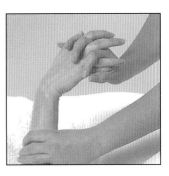

7 *With one hand make circular pressure movements round each of the three joints on each finger, starting at the tip. When you have worked round all three joints, gently rotate the finger twice. Then gently stretch each finger to release the joints.*

8 *Raising your partner's lower arm and supporting it with your left hand, clasp your partner's hand with your right hand, and gently rotate it in a half circle, three times in each direction.*

9 *Still supporting the lower arm, thread your fingers between your partner's and gently bend the wrist backward and forward three times, making sure that the wrist joint is not forced.*

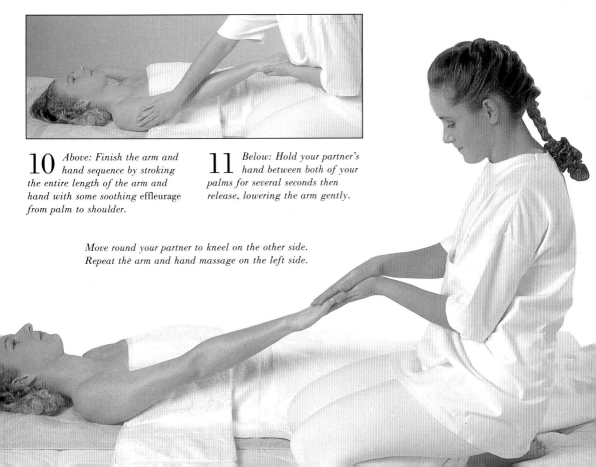

10 *Above: Finish the arm and hand sequence by stroking the entire length of the arm and hand with some soothing effleurage from palm to shoulder.*

11 *Below: Hold your partner's hand between both of your palms for several seconds then release, lowering the arm gently.*

Move round your partner to kneel on the other side. Repeat the arm and hand massage on the left side.

CHEST, SHOULDERS AND NECK

Ideally a chest massage should follow an arm massage and precede a facial massage. It's not only the hours spent sitting hunched over a desk that tighten and contract the chest muscles – clutching a car steering wheel, carrying heavy shopping, and poor posture all *have a cumulative effect. Tension in the chest can also exacerbate inflexibility and stiffness in the neck and the shoulders. We tend to raise the shoulders toward our ears, until they become set rigid with tension. This sequence includes work to help these problems.*

First check if your partner would be more comfortable with a small cushion or a folded towel under the head. They may or may not, but it is important that the neck should be comfortable. Kneel behind your partner's head to start the sequence.

CHEST

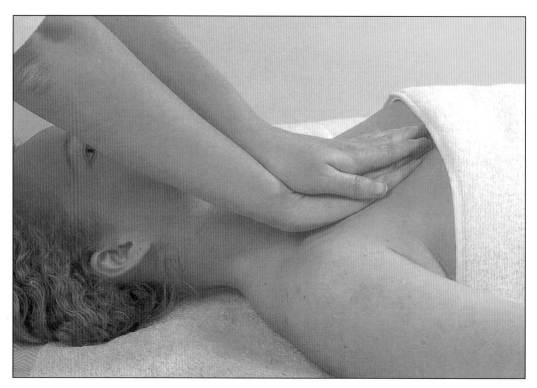

1 *Lightly oil the palm of your right hand, and with the flat of the hands placed on the chest, fingers pointing toward your* *partner's feet, place the left hand on top of the right. You will be doing reinforced* effleurage *on the right side of the chest first.*

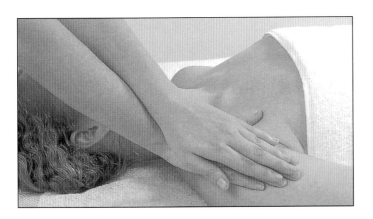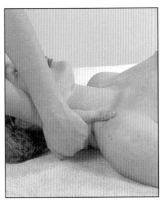

2 *Sweep your hands over the chest, toward and round the right shoulder, keeping the left hand over the right. The movement should be a continuous* effleurage *stroke. You should apply enough pressure to press the chest and shoulder toward the floor, so that they release as you lift off after the stroke. Repeat three times.*

3 *Continue the* effleurage *stroke, sweeping both hands round and up the right side of the neck.*

Repeat the sequence twice more, starting from the centre of the chest.

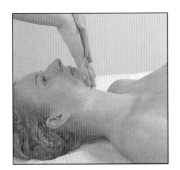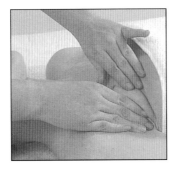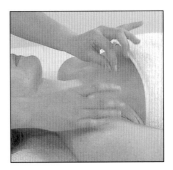

4 *Repeat the sequence once again, but this time finish by bringing both hands up to the jawline with the fingers resting lightly under the centre of the jaw.*

5 *With both hands, knead the fleshy area in front of the armpit. Pick up and release the muscles, squeezing them from one hand to the other.*

6 *On the same fleshy area, lightly pinch the surface muscles between the thumb and first finger. Alternate the hands swiftly in a rhythmical action, checking with your partner that there is no discomfort.*

Repeat the effleurage *strokes from the centre of the chest and over the right side of the neck in one continuous movement, to soothe the area you have worked on.*

Then repeat the entire sequence on the left side of the chest and neck, lightly oiling the palm of your left hand before you begin.

SHOULDERS AND NECK

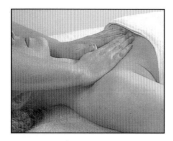

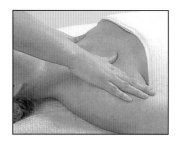

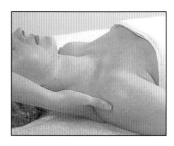

1 *Place both hands fairly firmly, side by side, over the front of the chest.*

2 *Sweep them out toward each shoulder with firm* effleurage *strokes, taking them over the shoulders, round under the upper back and up the back of the neck.*

3 *When you take the movement round the back and the neck gently lift the weight of your partner to give the muscles a gentle stretch.*

4 *Left: With the fingertips, work with circular pressures up the back of the neck to the base of the skull. These should be small, firm rotations, which you can feel easing taut muscles. You should spend some time on this area, which is often extremely tense.*

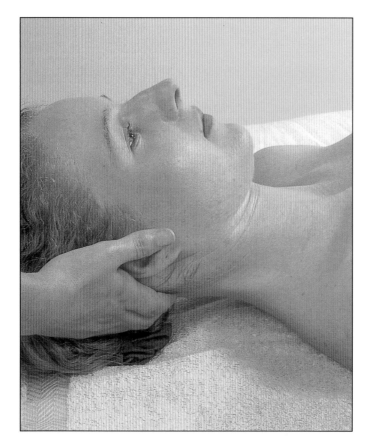

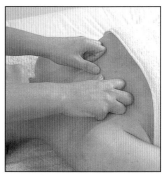

5 *With loose fists, use the knuckle area to ripple your fingers in semi-circular frictions all over the upper chest. Keep the half circles fairly small and apply quite firm pressure on the fleshier area, but avoid working directly on the collarbone.*

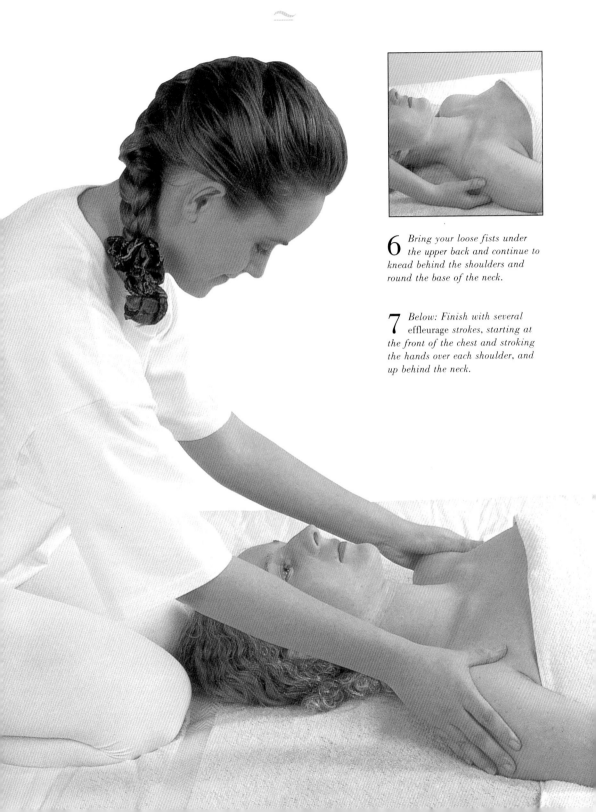

6 *Bring your loose fists under the upper back and continue to knead behind the shoulders and round the base of the neck.*

7 *Below: Finish with several effleurage strokes, starting at the front of the chest and stroking the hands over each shoulder, and up behind the neck.*

FACE

The face constantly mirrors our health and emotions. Stress and tension are reflected in a furrowed brow, and lines around the eyes, mouth and jawline. A face massage can soothe away headaches, anxiety and exhaustion and replace them with a feeling of serenity. It improves the circulation, giving the skin a healthy glow.

If your partner wears contact lenses make sure they are removed before you start a face massage. Use a little light facial oil, and don't let the oil get too near or in the eyes. Keep the hands relaxed. You may be surprised to find that the face is less fragile than it looks and you can apply quite deep pressure without discomfort.

Your partner will probably still prefer to have a small cushion or towel under the head. Use a towelling hairband to keep the hair off the face.

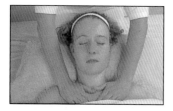
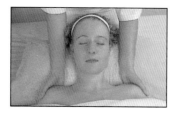
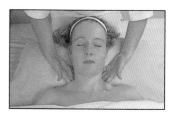

1 Kneel at the top of your partner's head and lightly oil your palms. With your hands placed over the collarbone, pointing away from you, get ready to begin some gentle effleurage strokes.

2 Sweep your hands out across the shoulders, keeping the pressure light.

3 In a continuous movement, bring your hands up round the back of the neck to the nape, pause for a moment, increasing the pressure slightly with the fingertips, then release and lift your hands away.

Repeat the effleurage sequence a minimum of three times.

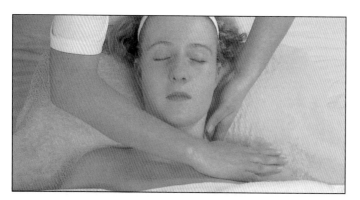
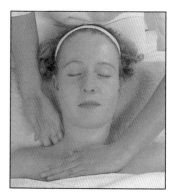

4 Bring your right arm across the front of your partner so the hand supports the left shoulder. Using light upward strokes, sweep your left hand up from the top of the shoulder, up the side of the neck to the edge of the jaw. Repeat three times.

5 Now repeat this movement on the other side of the neck.

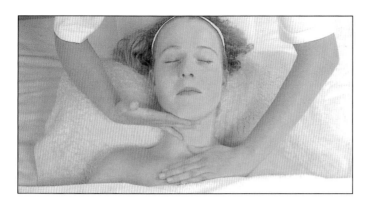

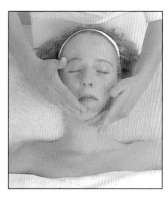

6 *Starting with both hands over the front of the chest, fingers pointing toward each other, lightly sweep the flat of one hand up the front of the neck to the jaw,*

flicking the hand away when you get there. As you flick the first hand away, bring the second up, so you stroke up with alternate hands. Repeat several times.

7 *Bring both hands up to the front of the jaw. Alternately sweep one hand and then the other up along the jawline toward the ear. Repeat several times.*

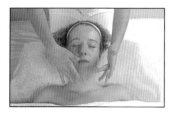

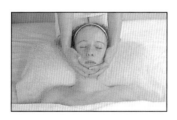

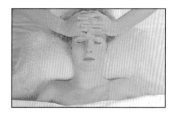

8 *Briskly tap the length of the jawline using the middle and ring fingers, starting from the centre front and working toward the ears. This should be a stimulating movement, so keep the patting quick and fairly firm.*

9 *Afterwards, soothe the area by cradling the face gently with both hands. Pause for several moments then release the hands.*

10 *Bring your hands up to the forehead. Loosely interlock your fingers, and using the palms apply gentle pressure over the forehead. Slowly unlock the fingers to release. Repeat three times.*

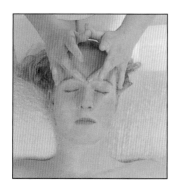

11 *Left: Starting with the third finger of each hand placed on the bridge of the nose, stroke out over the brows toward the temples at each side of the forehead. Come up the forehead a little and, starting again with both fingers at the centre front, repeat the strokes out toward the hairline.*

Repeat a couple of times more, bringing the fingers higher up the forehead each time, until the whole forehead is covered.

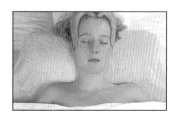

12 *To finish, place your hands on each side of your partner's head, and pause for a few seconds before lifting them away.*

ABDOMEN AND WAIST

Many people feel exposed and vulnerable when baring their abdomen so you will need to be particularly sensitive to your partner when it comes to this part of massage. Start with very gentle strokes, but try to be confident, as a gentle touch which is also tentative can feel unnerving for your partner.

Massage of the abdomen calms the nerves and can soothe stomach aches if they're caused by tension, poor digestion or period pains. It also stimulates the digestive organs so that elimination is improved. You should wait for at least an hour after your partner's meal before giving an abdominal massage.

Kneel beside your partner to do the massage. With a little practice you will find it is possible to tackle both sides from the same position. It helps to start and finish the massage by focusing on your partner's breathing so that your strokes coincide with the intake and expellation. To begin with, try slowly stroking your hands up from the lower abdomen to the chest on inhalation and down the sides on exhalation.

ABDOMEN

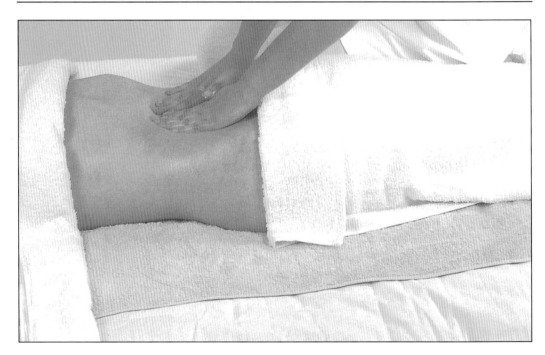

1 *Kneel beside your partner, level with the hips. Lightly oil the palms of the hands, and make contact by gently placing your* *hands together in a diamond shape over the lower abdomen, pointing toward the head. Keep the fingers together and the hands relaxed.* *Encourage your partner to breathe into the abdomen so you can feel it expand and contract. Work with the breath.*

122

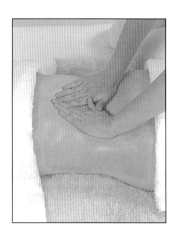

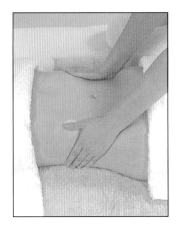

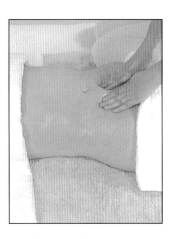

2 *Slowly slide your hands up the centre of the abdomen until you reach the ribs, making sure the pressure is even and not too firm.*

3 *Continue the movement by sweeping the hands out and round the sides of the waist. As you take them out from the ribs toward the sides you can apply a little more pressure, so that you feel the muscles being drawn outward.*

4 *Return to the starting position with both hands placed on the lower abdomen and repeat this continuous movement several times. Apply more oil as necessary.*

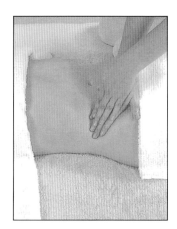

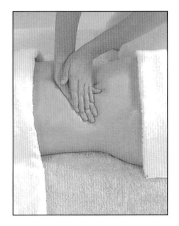

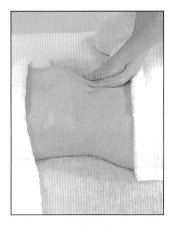

5 *Place both hands on your partner's lower abdomen at the right-hand side, ready to circle the navel. Your left hand rests over the right for support.*

6 *Stroke upward, keeping the left hand over the right, until you reach the ribs. The pressure can be quite firm to stimulate the digestive system. Keep the stroke smooth and continuous.*

7 *Continue the stroke by bringing your hands across under the ribs, and down the left side of your partner's abdomen. It is important that the direction you work in is up your partner's right side, across and down the left side.*

Repeat the navel-circling movement three times, each time returning to the centre of the lower abdomen.

WAIST

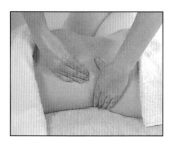

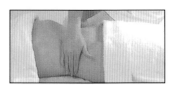

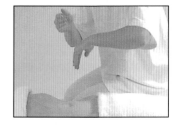

1 Begin kneading round the waist area by squeezing and releasing the flesh from one hand to the other. These movements should be firm and stimulating.

2,3 Right and below right: Cross your hands over your partner's waist so the palms are grasping the sides of the midriff. Briskly draw them up the side of the waist, uncrossing the hands over the top of the abdomen and turning the palms as they travel down the other side. Draw up again and recross the arms to the original starting position. Keep the speed of this fairly quick and apply firm pressure to draw the flesh up the sides, then lighten your touch across the top of the abdomen. Repeat four times.

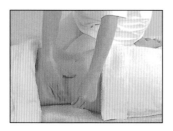

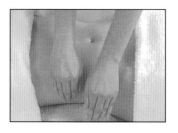

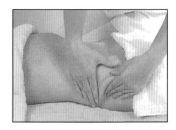

4 Starting at the far side of the waist, lightly pinch the flesh between fingers and thumbs with brisk, short stimulating movements. Repeat on the other side of the waist.

5 With loosely cupped hands, lightly cup the side of the waist, keeping the pace fast and stimulating, but at the same time checking that it is not causing discomfort. The action should be enough to increase the flow of blood to the area without hurting.

6 Working on the top of the hip area, squeeze and release the flesh in a kneading movement, using deep and stimulating pressure.

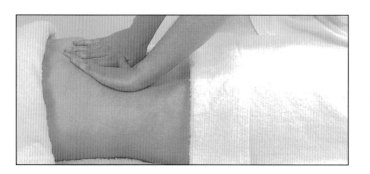

7 Left: Finish the massage of the abdomen by repeating the soothing effleurage strokes from the beginning of the sequence. End with both hands placed over the centre of the abdomen, fingers pointing toward the head. Hold for a few seconds before lifting off.

BACK OF BODY

Ask your partner to turn over on to their front, ready for you to start work on the back of the legs and buttocks. Rest their head to one side.

LEGS AND BUTTOCKS

The backs of the legs and buttocks offer plenty of scope for massage techniques. Most people can take plenty of firm massage on the larger muscles in the thighs and buttocks. The fleshy parts are ideal for kneading and squeezing and the firmer pressure can feel wonderfully satisfying. In contrast though, the most gentle effleurage can still stimulate other body functions to improve their efficiency. Poor circulation and a sluggish lymphatic system can be considerably improved with a good leg massage. Tiredness and heaviness in the legs is alleviated and your partner should have a renewed feeling of energy afterwards.

EFFLEURAGE

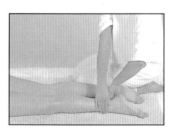

1 *Left: Start by kneeling on one side of your partner's ankles. You should be able to work on both legs from the same side. Begin by working on the leg furthest away from you.*
   Lightly oil your hands and place them crossed over the back of the left ankle.

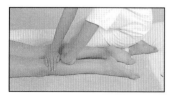

2 *In a smooth and continuous movement,* effleurage *up the leg, with right hand leading the left. When you get to the back of the knee pause for two seconds.*

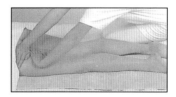

3 *Carry the stroke up the leg and at the top of the thigh cross the hands, keeping the pressure even and light.*

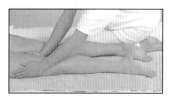

4 *Bring your hands back down the sides of the leg until you reach the back of the ankle again.*

Repeat the sequence three times, each time increasing the pressure slightly on the upward stroke toward the heart.

UPPER LEGS AND BUTTOCKS

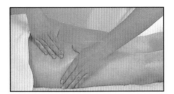

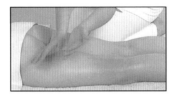

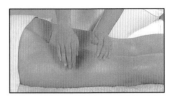

1 *Move to a kneeling position beside your partner's upper leg. Using a firm kneading movement, squeeze and release the back of the thigh muscles, working up to the buttocks. You should be able to pick up quite a large area of muscle between the hands.*

2 *With the outside edge of the hands, do some short sharp hacking movements. Alternate the hands in a quick, repetitive action. Continue the hacking all over the back of the upper leg and the buttocks.*

3 *Continue working on the upper leg and buttocks, with some cupping. The cupping action should be short and fast to stimulate the whole area.*

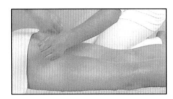

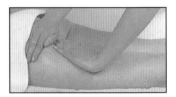

4 *With loose fists, briskly pound the top and outside of the thigh. You can use the backs of your fingers or the outside edge of the fists. Use a firmer knuckling action over the buttock area.*

5 *Follow this sequence of friction movements with soothing effleurage strokes from the back of the knee to the top of the thigh, sweeping out and back down the leg to the knee.*

CALVES

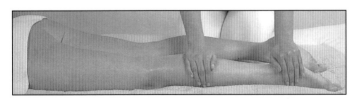

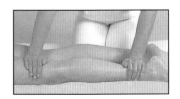

1 *Move back down to kneel beside your partner's ankles. Lightly oil your hands again if necessary. Start with both hands on the back of your partner's ankle. Smooth your right hand up toward the knee, keeping your left hand on the ankle for support.*

2 *Continue to stroke the right hand toward the thigh, keeping the pressure light as you reach the back of the knee.*

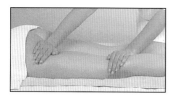 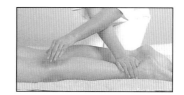 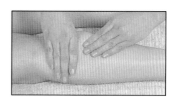

3 As you continue the stroke, taking your right hand up toward the top of the thigh, simultaneously slide your left hand up the lower leg to the back of the knee. Try to make this a flowing movement.

4 Without pausing, bring your right hand in a continuous stroke back down the leg. When you reach the knee you will need to slide the left hand off the knee, so the right hand can continue right down to the ankle again.

5 Start kneading the calf with both hands, working from the ankle up to the knee. Don't knead the back of the knee. Squeeze and release the calf muscle as you go. If your partner's calf muscles are particularly tight this kneading action may feel uncomfortable, so ask your partner if the pressure is right.

Repeat three times, or until you feel confident with the movement.

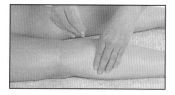 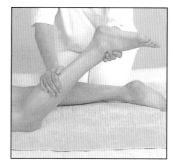 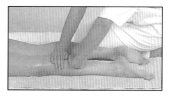

6 Do some short, sharp pinching movements all over the calf muscle, again checking that you are not hurting your partner.

7 Left: Lifting and supporting your partner's leg in the left hand, slide your right hand up from the back of the ankle to the knee. Keep the pressure as firm as is comfortable. Repeat three times. Gently return the leg to rest on the floor.

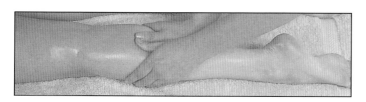

8 With your thumbs together start at the back of the ankle, and work up the back of the calf to the knee, applying pressure firm enough to release tightness in these muscles. When you reach the back of the knee, lighten the pressure and sweep your hands back down the sides of the leg to the ankle. Repeat three times.

9 To complete the back of the leg massage, repeat the effleurage strokes from the beginning of the sequence, stroking the leg from ankle to thigh and back down to the ankle again. Repeat three times to soothe the leg.

Repeat the entire back of leg massage on your partner's other leg, covering the leg you have worked on with a towel to keep the muscles warm.

BACK AND SHOULDERS

The back is an area of great strength and mobility, and it is the main supportive structure of the body. It therefore warrants more attention than most other areas. By working on the back you can reach nerves affecting every part of the body.

Full back massage, with emphasis on the spine and lower back, greatly alleviates effects of stress throughout the body, enhancing physical and psychological well-being. Smooth, flowing strokes stretch the muscles and tissues round contours of the back, and help restore flexibility for health and mobility, whilst stronger strokes along the spinal muscles and over the lower back bring deeper relief to aching or knotted muscles.

You should never massage directly on the spine itself, although working down each side is highly beneficial. Avoid using percussion strokes such as hacking and cupping on the kidneys, which are level with the waistline in the centre of the back.

First, make sure your partner is comfortable, lying face down with arms resting beside the face. Support the forehead with a rolled towel, and if helpful, use a pillow, cushion or rolled towel under the chest. It helps to have hair clear from the back of the neck.

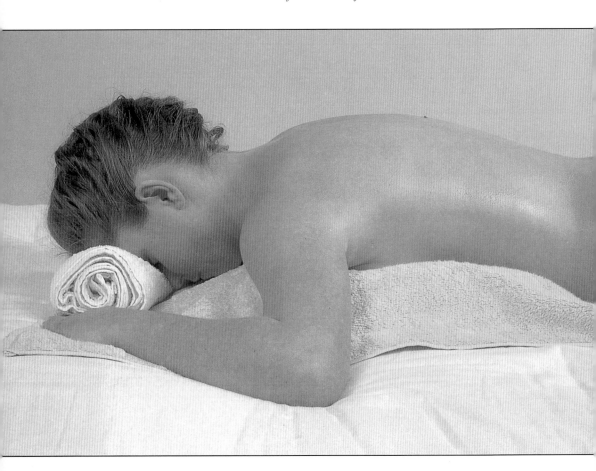

EFFLEURAGE

Kneel beside your partner's right hip and oil your hands. With your first long effleurage *strokes try to concentrate on finding areas of particular tension and tightness.*

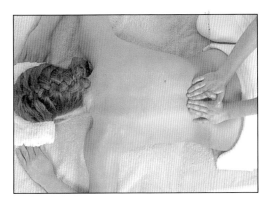

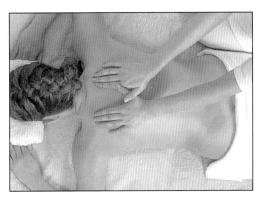

1 *Starting at the lower back begin the* effleurage *strokes. With thumbs crossed to connect the hands together, move slowly up the centre of the back, putting firm pressure on the fingertips.*

2 *Take the stroke up to the top of the back in a continuous movement.*

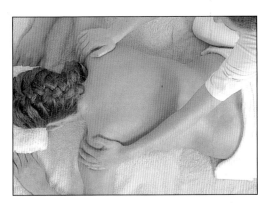

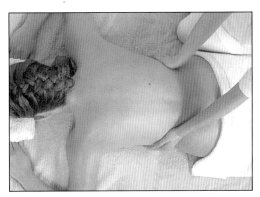

3 *Without a pause, separate the hands at the top of the back, sweeping them out and round the shoulders.*

4 *Continue the stroke, bringing both hands down the sides of the back to the lower back, ready to begin again.*

Repeat this effleurage *sequence three times, oiling your hands each time.*

SHOULDERS

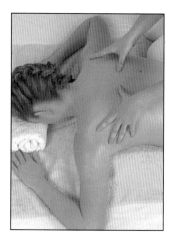

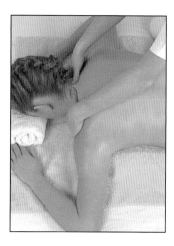

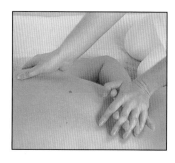

3 Carefully bring your partner's arm across the hollow of the back and clasp their right hand with your left to support the arm. The shoulder blade should now stick out slightly. With your right thumb make circular pressure movements over the shoulder area. Strong muscles support the shoulder blade and you can work firmly under the bone itself to release tightness in this area.

1 Using your thumbs each side of the spine, start level with the shoulder blades and make circling pressure movements, working quite firmly into the muscles.

2 Continue working up each side of the spine until you reach the nape of the neck.

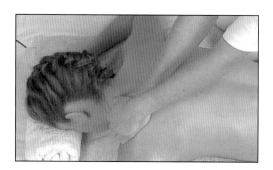

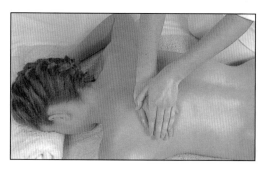

4 With your left hand resting over your right to increase the pressure, work in small, circular movements from the base of the neck out over the shoulder.

5 Continue round to the shoulder blade, using firm pressure to release tension in the muscle.

Move to the other side of your partner and repeat these steps on the other shoulder.

BACK

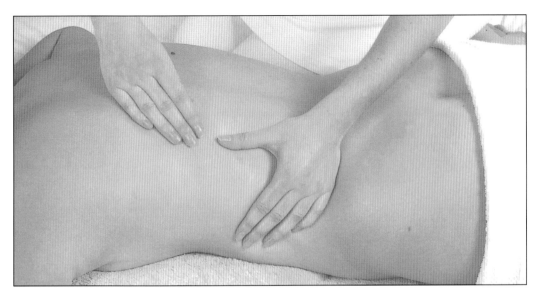

1 *Kneeling to the right side of your partner, start to knead the far side of the back firmly with both hands, beginning at the outer* sides of the waist. Pick up, roll and release the muscles, alternately pressing one hand toward another. Continue kneading up the back *until you reach the shoulders. Start again at the waist but this time come closer to the spine and repeat the line of kneading up the back.*

Repeat the kneading on the near side of the back. You should be able to do this without moving your kneeling position.

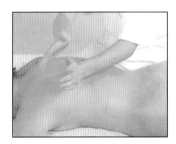

2 *Using the outer edge of the hands, briskly and rhythmically hack from the lower back up to the shoulders, but avoid the bony shoulder blade. Try to visualize each side of the back divided into three sections, so you cover the whole back thoroughly.*

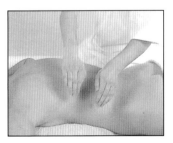

3 *Start cupping from the lower back up the back and across the shoulders. The action should be quick, with alternate hands striking the back briskly.*

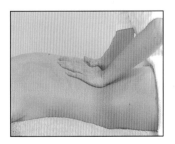

4 *Repeat the effleurage strokes from the beginning of the sequence to soothe the back. Repeat a number of times.*

SPINE

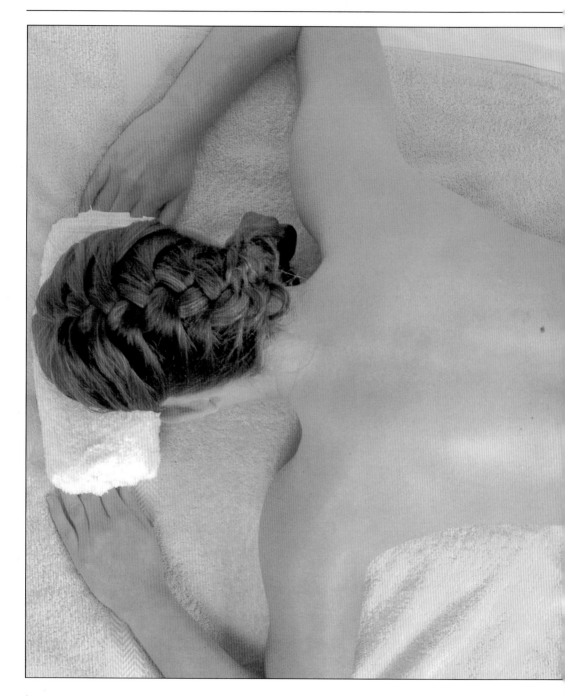

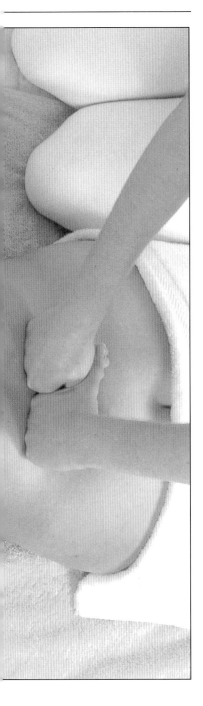

1 *Left: With loose fists, and thumbs crossed for support, push the top of the hands up each side of the spine to the nape of the neck.*

2 *Right: Uncurl the fingers when you get to the nape and sweep them back down the sides of the back. Repeat three times.*

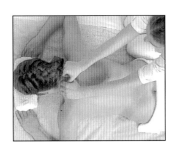

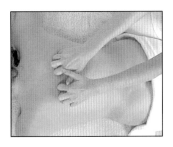

3 *Starting at the lower back, place the thumbs on either side of the spine, resting your hands either side of the back. Rotate the thumbs in small circles, travelling up the sides of the spine until you reach the hairline. Use firm pressure. Reverse the movement, circling your thumbs back down each side of the spine.*

4 *Starting at the lower back, use loose knuckles, crossing your thumbs over each other for support, to work up either side of the spine and back down again. Repeat twice.*

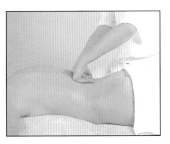

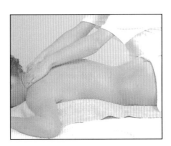

5 *Using the backs of your hands and starting at the lower back, push up either side of the spine to just above the waistline. Then sweep your hands outward and back down round the hips. Repeat three times.*

6 *To finish the massage, repeat the effleurage strokes from the beginning of the sequence, starting at the lower back, up the back, round the shoulders and down again to the lower back, in a continuous sweeping movement.*

SELF MASSAGE

A simple, effective self massage can do wonders to ease away tension and restore energy after a stressful, tiring day. After a shower or bath, massaging the body with lotions and oils is very relaxing and helps keep the skin in glowing condition.

You can use self massage to target particular aches and pains or areas of tension, for relief just where you need it. The beauty of self massage is you can do it to suit your needs and moods at any time – to unwind in the evening or to energize yourself in the morning.

SHOULDERS

1 *Sitting upright, start from the base of the neck and press down with your fingers along the top of the shoulders. As you reach the bony part of the shoulder, slide your hand back to the base of the neck, and repeat the pressing at least three times. Finish by stroking firmly from neck to shoulder and then repeat on the other side of the neck.*

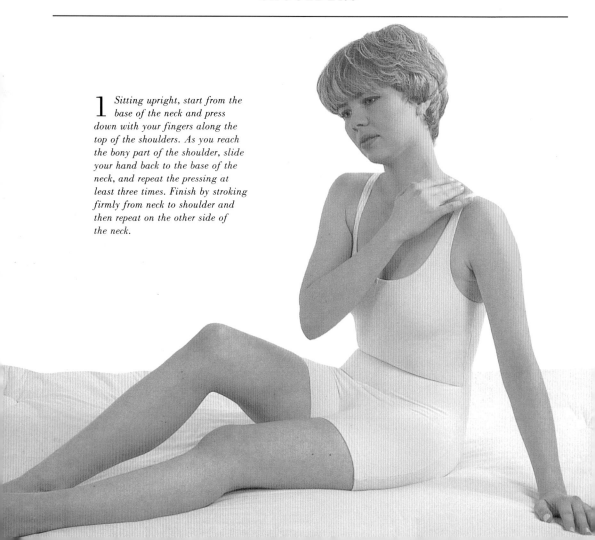

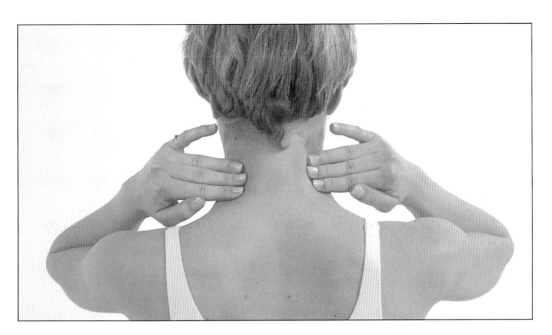

2 Use the fingertips of both hands to make small circular movements, working up the back of the neck. Gentle circular movements, where you can feel yourself easing muscular tightness, are better than direct, static pressures on this area. Continue up and round the base of the skull.

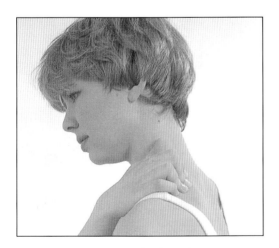

3 Knead each shoulder with a firm squeezing action, rolling the flesh between your fingers and the ball of the hand. Repeat several times on each side.

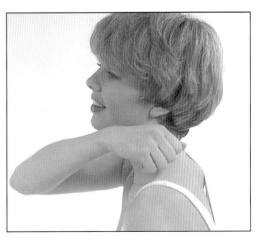

4 With your hand in a loose fist, pummel your shoulder lightly, keeping the wrist and elbow relaxed. Use light, springy movements to stimulate the area. Repeat on the other shoulder.

ARMS

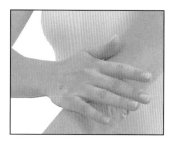

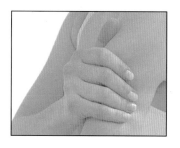

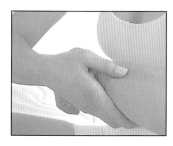

1 *Stroke firmly up the arm from the wrist to the shoulder, returning with a lighter touch. Repeat the stroke several times on different parts of the arm.*

2 *Pressing your fingers toward the palm of the hand, knead up the arm from the elbow to the shoulder. Cover the area thoroughly, working right round the arm.*

3 *Starting from the wrist, knead up the forearm toward the elbow, this time using your thumb to make circular movements.*

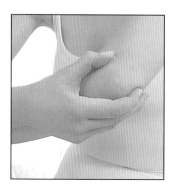

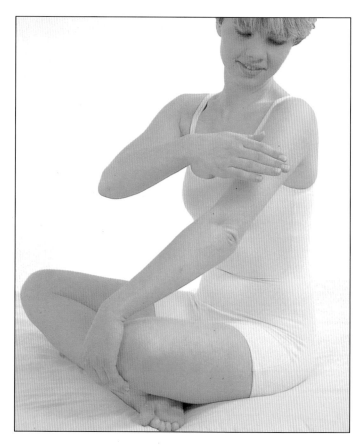

4 *With thumb and fingers make circular pressures round the elbow. First, work round the far side of the elbow with your working arm coming over the top of the arm you're massaging, then bend that arm up and work from the inside of your elbow. You may need more oil for dry elbows.*

5 *Right: Gently but briskly pat your upper arm, or use some gentle cupping. Follow with some effleurage stroking up and down the whole arm again to finish. Work on the hand before massaging the other arm.*

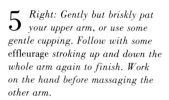

HANDS

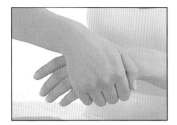

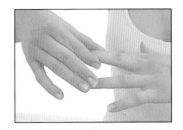

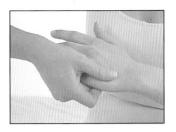

1 *Squeeze the hand firmly, spreading the palm laterally. Cover the whole of the hand, fingers and wrist.*

2 *Using circular pressure, squeeze each finger joint between your finger and thumb. Then hold the base of each finger and pull the finger gently to stretch it, sliding your grip up to the top of the finger in a continuous movement.*

3 *With circular thumb pressures, work up each of the furrows between the bones in the hand, from the knuckle to the wrist. When you have covered each furrow, smooth the hand by stroking.*

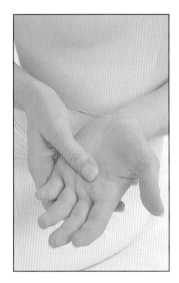

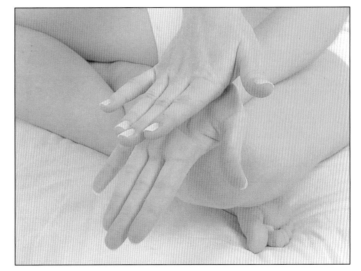

4 *Turn the hand over to work on the palm. Cover the area with circular thumb pressures, paying particular attention to the heel of the hand and the wrist. Follow this with some deeper, static pressures all over the palm.*

5 *Finish by stroking the palm of one hand with the other. This can be quite a firm stroke, working from the tips of the fingers to the wrist, leading with the pressure*

from the heel of the hand. Stroke back to the fingers and repeat twice more, each time using slightly less pressure. Finally, stroke the inside of the wrist.

Repeat the whole of the arm and hand massage sequences on the other side.

BACK AND ABDOMEN

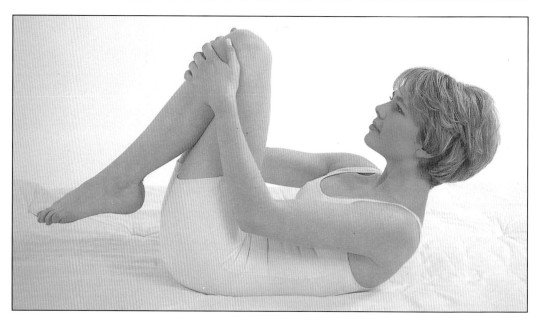

1 *Lie on your back, clasp your knees and gently rock backward and forward to massage* the lower back, buttocks and hip joints and gently stretch out the vertebrae.

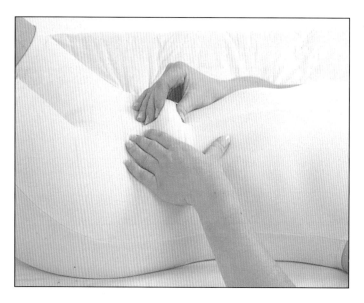

2 *Left: Bend your knees up and use some gentle* petrissage *to knead the whole of the abdominal area. When you have finished kneading, place both hands flat on the centre of the abdomen, fingers pointing slightly together, and pause for a few moments. Then smooth your hands outward over the hips and thighs in a long, slow, moulding movement.*

BUTTOCKS, HIPS AND THIGHS

1 *Kneel up and pummel your hips and buttocks, using a clenched fist and keeping your wrists flexible.*

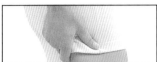

2 *With the thumb and fingers, squeeze and release the muscles firmly and slowly, working from the top of the thigh over the buttock. Repeat on the left side.*

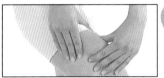

3 *Use both hands to squeeze and release the muscles on the front and side of the thigh, kneading the entire upper leg. Repeat on the other side.*

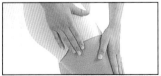

4 *Starting at the knee, stroke up the thigh with both hands to soothe the leg.*

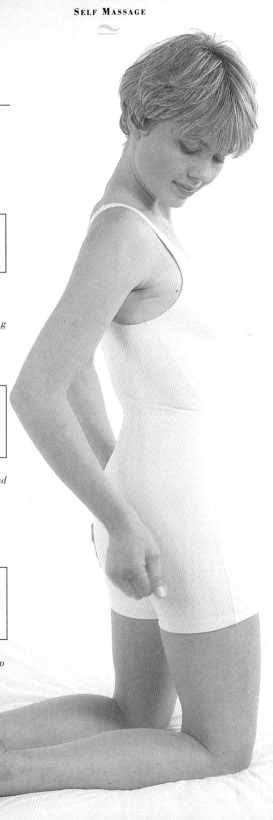

LEGS

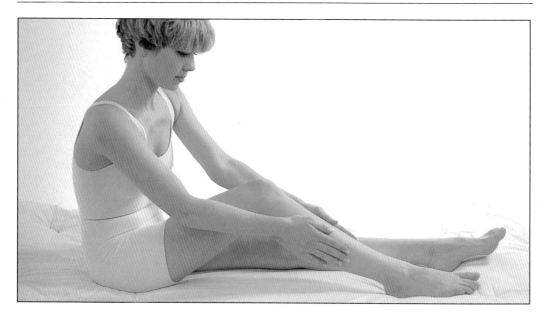

1 *Sitting down, with one leg raised slightly, stroke the leg with both hands from ankle to thigh. Begin the stroke as close to the ankle as you can reach. Repeat several times, moving round the leg slightly each time to stroke a different part.*

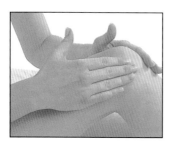

2 *Massage the knee, stroking round the outside of the kneecap to begin with, then using circular pressure with the fingertips to work round the kneecap more firmly.*

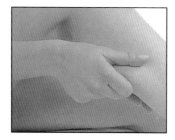

3 *Knead the calf muscle with both hands, using a firm petrissage to loosen any tension in the muscle.*

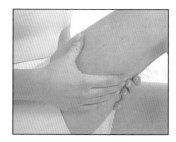

4 *Continue the kneading on the thigh, working over the top and outside areas with alternate hands. Whilst the leg is still raised, do some soothing effleurage strokes up the back of the leg from ankle to hip.*

Continue with the foot massage (opposite) before repeating all the steps on the other leg.

FEET

1 *Sitting down and leaning back, raise a leg, supporting the weight with your hands. Rotate the right ankle five times in each direction.*

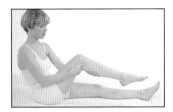

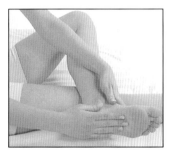

2 *Gently bring your foot over the other leg. With one hand on top of the foot and one underneath, stroke up the foot from toes to ankle. Repeat three times.*

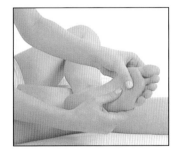

3 *With the thumbs, apply circular pressure over the ball of the foot. Work in lines from the inside of the foot to the outer edge. Repeat three times.*

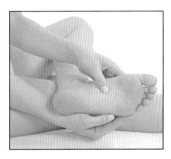

4 *Supporting the foot with one hand, continue the circular pressures over the raised instep, working from the inner to the outer edge. Repeat three times.*

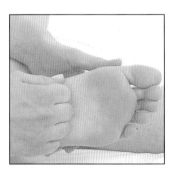

5 *Still holding the foot with one hand, make a loose fist with the other and firmly rotate your fist over the instep. Work thoroughly into the arch.*

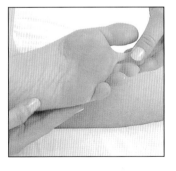

6 *Massage each toe individually. Slowly stretch the toe between the thumb and finger, pull gently, moving your fingers up the toe each time, until you reach the tip.*

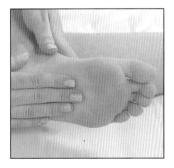

7 *Repeat the effleurage strokes of the foot, with one hand over and one under the foot, working from toes to ankle, several times.*

Repeat the leg and foot massage sequence on the other side.

MASSAGE AND EXERCISE

Professional sports people value massage very highly, not least because it works on several levels. Used before exercise it can prepare the body for the increase in activity not only by warming and loosening the muscles and joints (increasing their flexibility and helping to prevent cramp and injuries), but also by stimulating the system, both physically and mentally. This is the key to improved performance. After an exercise session, massage speeds up the elimination of waste products (in particular lactic acid) by stimulating the lymphatic system. The accumulation of these waste products during exercise is the cause of much of the stiffness and pain experienced afterwards.

STRAINS AND SPRAINS

A burning sensation under the skin is likely to indicate that muscles, fibres or ligaments have been strained – stretched beyond their natural limits. This is often the result of exercising without an adequate warm-up routine or over-exertion. A routine of pre-exercise massage and limbering will help to prevent strains. Gently massaging the affected area will also help to speed recovery.

Sprains are more serious and are caused by violent wrenching of a joint, most commonly the ankle, wrist or knee. The surrounding muscles, ligaments and tendons may also be damaged and the affected area may be extremely painful and swollen. Apply an ice-pack or cold compress for 15–20 minutes to reduce the swelling. When it is removed you can start to massage the area gently (as shown opposite), taking care not to work directly on the swelling. Rest the ankle as much as possible and use a support bandage.

A serious sprain should always be checked by a doctor in case a bone has been fractured, and a sprained knee always requires medical attention.

CRAMP

You don't have to be a fitness fanatic to suffer from cramp. On the contrary, it is usually underused or ill-prepared muscles which go into cramp. It doesn't even take movement to set it off: the searing pain of cramp can occur in the middle of the night, when the reduced circulation has caused muscles to contract. Frequent cramps may indicate generally poor circulation or a deficiency of calcium or salt. Massage will increase the blood circulation to alleviate the pain. You should also try to stretch out the affected muscle.

BACKACHE

Back strain is the most common source of debilitating pain. Most sports put increased strain on the legs, buttocks and back. Previous injuries can make the back prone to recurrent pain. Awkward, inappropriate or excessive exercise can also cause trouble. You should never subject the back to unnecessary strain. With regular and thorough back massage (particularly before exercise) the likelihood of injury is reduced. If, however, you want a quick warm-up for the back, or an after-exercise sequence, follow the instant back and shoulder massage. Always consult a doctor, osteopath or chiropractor if in any doubt about the seriousness of a back problem.

WITH OR WITHOUT OILS

You don't always have to oil at hand, and it certainly isn't crucial for massaging unexpected strains, sprains and cramps. If you do have some light vegetable oil nearby, all the better, but don't worry if you don't.

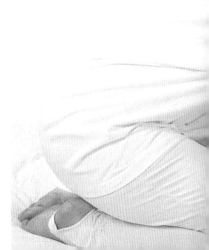

ANKLE STRAIN OR SPRAIN

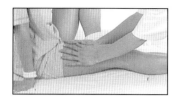 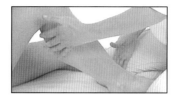 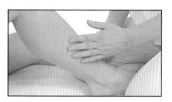

1 *Above and below: Avoid working directly on the swollen area. Start with gentle* effleurage *strokes working from the knee toward the thigh. Massaging in the direction of the lymph nodes in the groin will help drain away the fluids that have accumulated round the joint. Lightly stroke back to the knee. Repeat several times.*

2 *Help your partner to bend the affected leg. Continue the* effleurage *strokes on the lower leg, this time working from the ankle to the knee, alternating your hands. Repeat several times, then gently squeeze the calves with one hand, with the other supporting the foot.*

3 *Concentrating on the ankle area, stroke extremely gently all round the ankle with short upward movements. Check that this is not causing discomfort.*

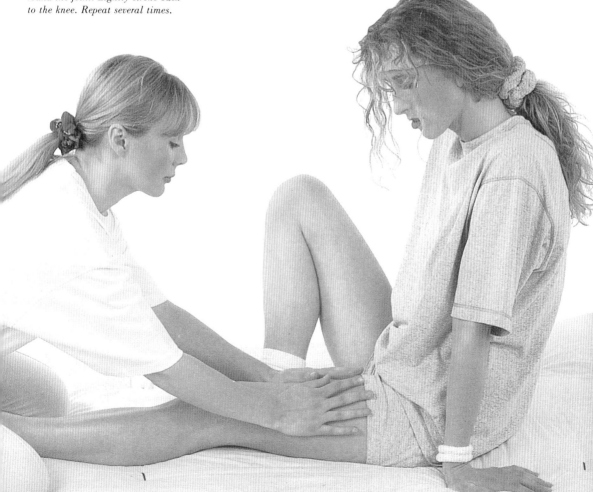

CALF CRAMP

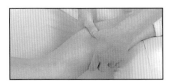

1. *With your partner lying face down and the foot supported across your leg or a small pillow, gradually apply direct thumb pressure into the belly of the cramped calf muscle for eight to ten seconds.*

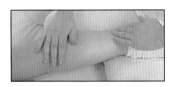

2. *Do some* effleurage *strokes, working from ankle to thigh and back down again.*

SELF-HELP STRETCH

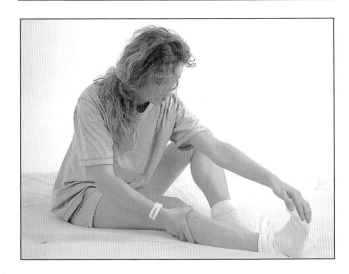

A good way of dealing with calf cramp is to sit down with the affected leg straight and stretch the toes toward you. Hold this position for eight seconds and then release. Repeat a few times, until the spasm seems to be lessening. Then knead your calf muscle using firm pressure. When the muscle feels more relaxed switch to effleurage *strokes, working up the leg.*

HAMSTRING CRAMP

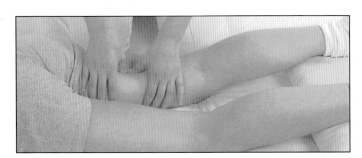

1. *With your partner lying face down and the ankles raised on a small pillow or cushion, begin massaging up the back of the thigh using alternate hands in slow, rhythmical stroking movements. Then apply static pressure to the middle of the thigh with the thumbs, holding for eight to ten seconds.*

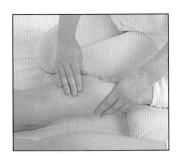

2. *Firmly knead the calf muscle. Squeeze, press and release the muscle using one hand after the other. Finally, do some soothing* effleurage *strokes up from ankle to thigh and back down again.*

HAMSTRING SELF-HELP STRETCH

Lie down flat, with the affected leg raised and the other knee bent. Stretch the muscle by pulling the thigh gently toward the chest.

Then firmly stroke up the back of your thigh for eight to ten seconds. Start to knead the back of the thigh until you feel the muscles begin to relax. Finally stroke over the area to soothe it.

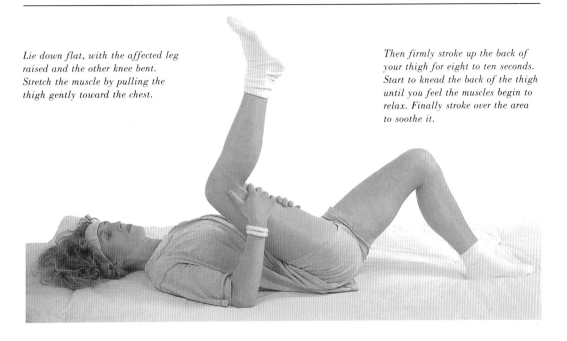

TENNIS OR GOLFER'S ELBOW

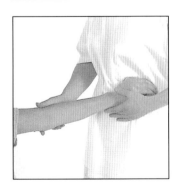

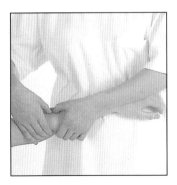

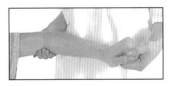

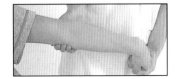

1 Support your partner's wrist in one hand and use soothing *effleurage* strokes along both sides of the arm, stroking from the wrist to the elbow and back again. Repeat several times.

2 Rest your partner's hand against your side. Continue working up from the wrist to the elbow and back, making small circular movements with both thumbs, paying particular attention to the muscles in the forearm.

3, 4 Secure your partner's hand in yours, and with the other hand supporting the elbow, flex the elbow forward, bringing the hand back to give the tendons that attach to the bones a good stretch.

BABY MASSAGE

A newborn baby instinctively responds to touch, and massage between mother and baby is a marvellous way of enhancing the natural bonding. All babies have this powerful sensitivity to being caressed and cuddled. Watch how a baby tightly curls its hands or toes as soon as something touches them.

There is no fixed sequence for massaging a baby. Keep the movements gentle and flowing. The simple action of gently stroking a baby will strengthen the natural bonding, and soothe and reassure the baby too. Massage has been shown to help calm difficult or colicky babies, and alleviate wind and other digestive problems. It may also build resistence to coughs and colds. Use a little light vegetable oil which is easily absorbed, such as sweet almond or sunflower, taking care to avoid the eyes.

GETTING COMFORTABLE

Lay the baby gently on the back on a warm, soft towel between your legs, or on your lap, whichever is most comfortable. Pour about 1 teaspoon (5 ml) of sweet almond oil into a small dish. Make sure your hands are warm and that the room is quiet, very warm and there are no draughts. After a baby's bathtime is ideal.

WORKING ON BABY'S FRONT

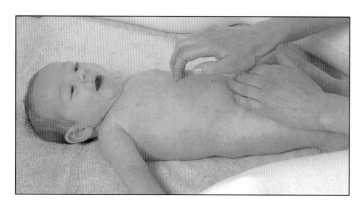

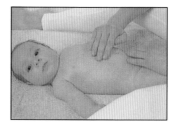

2 *Keeping the pressure very light, smooth both hands over the abdomen in continuous circular strokes, working up the baby's right side, across and down the baby's left side. Keep the movement continuous by lifting your left hand when your arms cross. Repeat these circular strokes several times.*

1 *Slowly and gently, smooth a little of the oil all over the front of the baby's body, shoulders to feet, avoiding the face. Lightly* *stroke down the chest and abdomen, with the tips of your fingers. This is a delightful stroke which can be used to calm a baby anytime.*

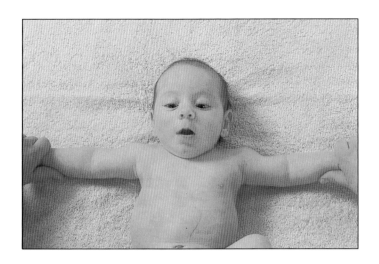

3 *Left: Gently stretch out both arms to the side, spreading the hands and fingers if the baby will let you. Gently squeeze out along the arms, then massage the wrist and palms with light, circular thumb movements. Finish by stretching out each finger with a slight pull.*

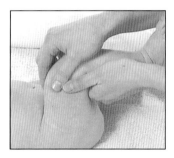

4 *Move on to the legs and feet, working on one leg at a time. Support the leg with both hands and gently squeeze and release the fleshy part of the thigh. Then, supporting the leg with one hand, stroke the leg from the knee to the thigh and back down again.*

5 *Right: Move your supporting hand down to behind the ankle. Gently smooth the palm of your other hand over the top of the foot from toe to ankle and back again. When you get to the toes, very gently stretch each one in turn.*

Repeat steps 4 and 5 on the baby's other leg.

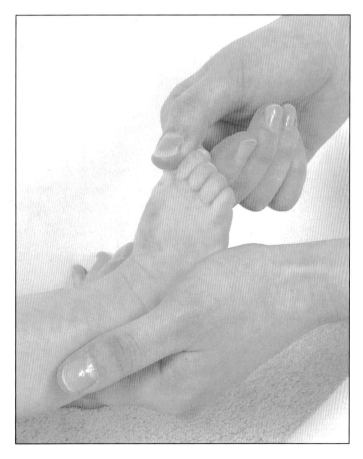

WORKING ON BABY'S BACK

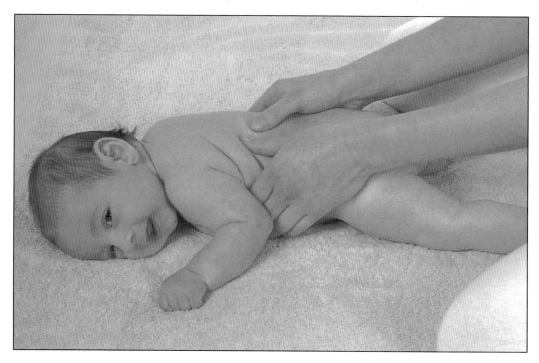

1 *Turn the baby over on to the front. Begin by stroking up the whole back to distribute a little oil.* *Take your strokes round the sides as well and then up the legs, back and out over the arms. Gentle* *massage on the back like this is particularly soothing because of its calming effect on the spinal nerves.*

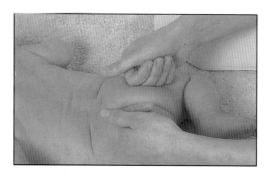

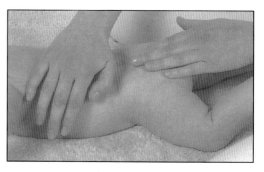

2 *Gently knead and squeeze the buttocks to stimulate the circulation. Make a loose fist and rotate over the buttocks, in circular movements.*

3 *Alternating your hands, one over the other, gently stroke up one side of the back to the shoulders and down again. Repeat on the other side of the back.*

4 *Bring both hands round the sides of the upper body, and use your thumbs to massage gently up the back to the base of the neck, and down again. Include some gentle massage with the thumbs on the shoulders.*

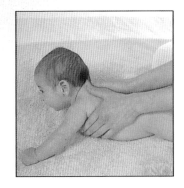

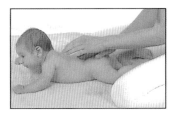

5 *To finish, repeat the feather strokes used at the beginning of the massage, working all over the back from neck to buttocks.*

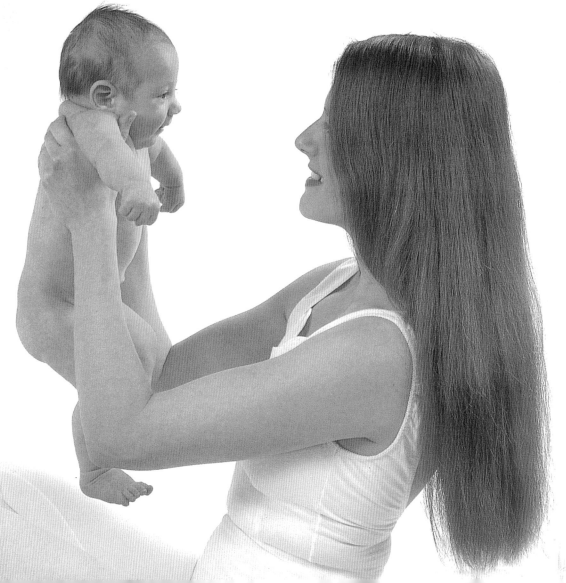

MASSAGE FOR OLDER PEOPLE

As we get older, painful, stiff joints, rheumatism and other signs of wear and tear become all too common. There are many ways to minimize the discomfort that the aging process brings. Good nutrition and remaining as active as possible are as crucial as ever, and massage can help in reducing pain, alleviating stiffness and retaining mobility. Increasing the blood circulation and gently releasing stiffness and inflexibility, it is a good way to help keep active. It isn't necessary to lie down – sitting on a chair is fine for massage of the neck and shoulders, and you can raise the leg on a stool for a leg, foot and ankle massage.

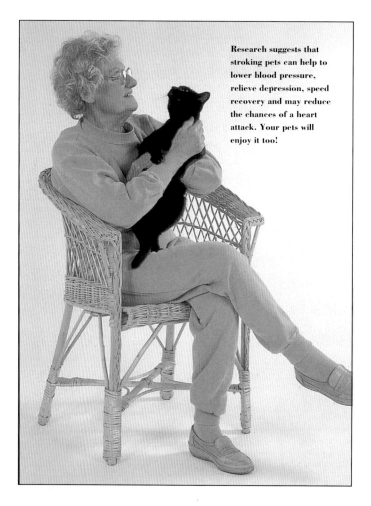

Research suggests that stroking pets can help to lower blood pressure, relieve depression, speed recovery and may reduce the chances of a heart attack. Your pets will enjoy it too!

Many older people suffer from aches and pains brought on by cold damp weather. A warm bath using aromatic essential oils such as lavender or sandalwood can comfort, soothe and relax you. Follow the bath with a gentle massage, and you will make headway in practising self-help. Massage stiff joints such as at wrists, knees, ankles and the hip. If the joint is affected by rheumatoid arthritis, massaging above and below the swollen area can relieve pain by relaxing the surrounding muscles. Avoid any swollen or inflamed areas.

The general wear and tear of joints which comes with aging is called osteoarthritis, and usually affects hips and knees in particular. Because the pain is often caused by the surrounding muscles, rather than the joint itself, massage can help to soothe the spasm and relieve pain. So long as the area is not swollen or inflamed you can massage the joint itself, working gently into the area which hurts most.

Massage can help to fulfil the deep-seated need for touch and communication, bringing psychological as well as physiological benefits, and contributing to a well-balanced lifestyle.

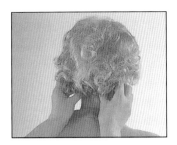

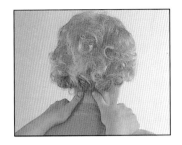

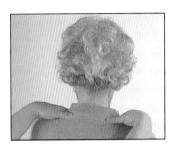

1 Start by gently resting your thumbs on the base of your partner's skull, just under the bony part. Relax your hands round each side of the head. Slowly and without too much pressure, slide your thumbs up through the hair, until you get halfway up the back of the head. Repeat three times, from the base of the skull to halfway up the head, to stimulate the nervous system.

2 Place the thumbs on the back of the neck and press gently, starting at the base of the skull and working down in a straight line toward the shoulders. This will loosen stiffness and relieve tension in the area. Repeat three times down the centre each time.

3 With your hand on either side of the neck, gently knead the tops of the shoulders, squeezing and releasing the muscles between your thumbs and fingers. Repeat three times the full length of the shoulder.

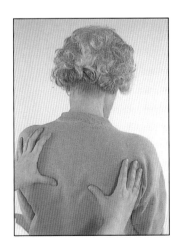

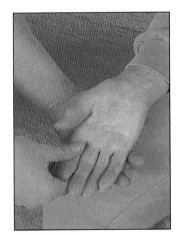

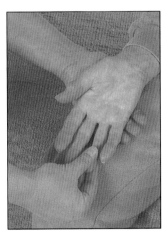

4 Bring your hands lower down the back near each shoulder blade, and use thumbs and fingers to massage upward over the shoulder blades, right up to the top of the shoulders. Slightly push into the back and release. Repeat from start to finish three times. You can vary the movement slightly by rotating the fingers as you work up.

5 Use any of the massage or self-massage techniques for the hands or feet, but avoid working directly on any joints inflamed with arthritis. Work above and below a swelling and then stroke up the limb toward the nearest lymph node. This stimulates the elimination of waste products and reduces inflammation.

6 If there are no signs of inflammation, you can use circular thumb movements all over the palm, then turn the hand over and work along each finger to the tip. Gently stretch each joint as far as it will go without causing pain, and then soothe the whole hand with firm strokes toward the wrist.

THE SENSUAL TOUCH

In the right circumstances, with a softly lit room, relaxing music, and using some of the more aphrodisiac essential oils such as rose, patchouli, neroli or sandalwood, a massage can be a highly pleasurable and sensual experience, relaxing the body and arousing the senses. Intuition will play a larger part in a sensual massage, as you discover which areas have the strongest impact on your partner's senses. It certainly isn't just the most obvious erogenous zones that bring pleasure – the back of the neck, scalp, solar plexus, inside of the elbows, hands and feet are just a few others.

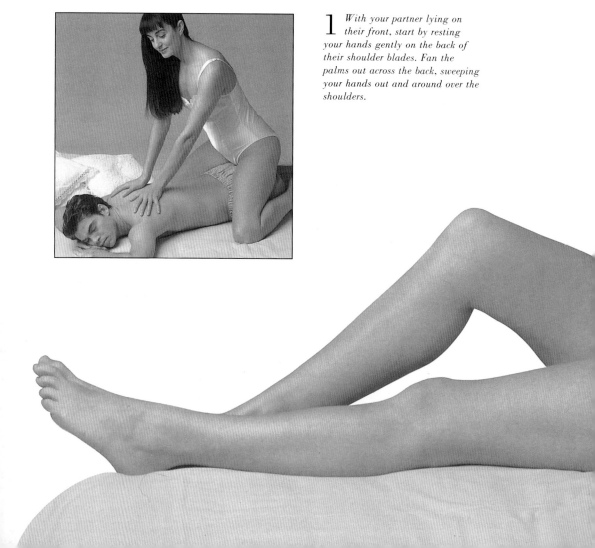

1 *With your partner lying on their front, start by resting your hands gently on the back of their shoulder blades. Fan the palms out across the back, sweeping your hands out and around over the shoulders.*

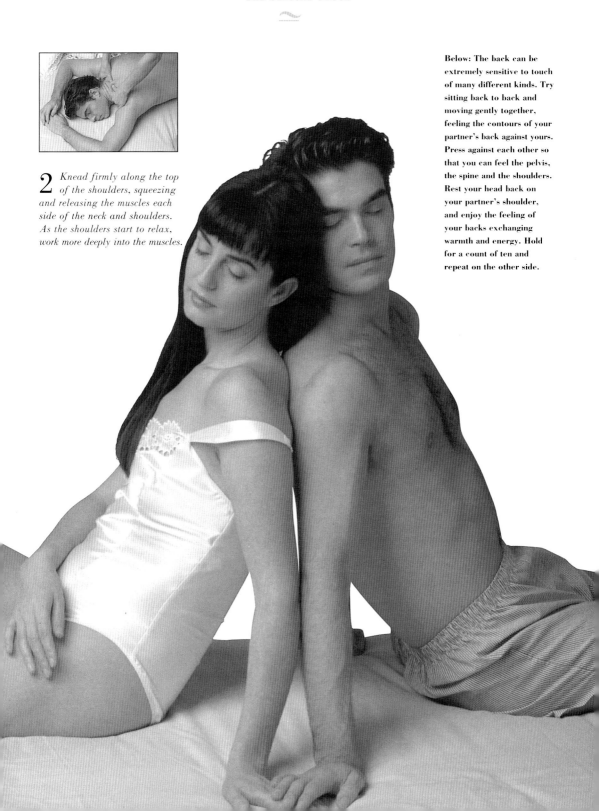

2 *Knead firmly along the top of the shoulders, squeezing and releasing the muscles each side of the neck and shoulders. As the shoulders start to relax, work more deeply into the muscles.*

Below: The back can be extremely sensitive to touch of many different kinds. Try sitting back to back and moving gently together, feeling the contours of your partner's back against yours. Press against each other so that you can feel the pelvis, the spine and the shoulders. Rest your head back on your partner's shoulder, and enjoy the feeling of your backs exchanging warmth and energy. Hold for a count of ten and repeat on the other side.

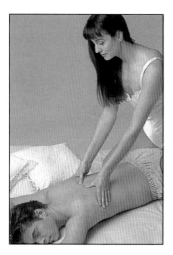 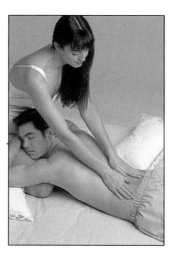 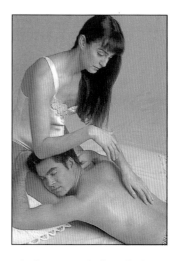

3 Check that your partner's head is still comfortable, then beginning at the nape of the neck let your thumbs gently stroke down each side of the spine. When you get to the lower back return up each side of the spine, this time working with slightly more pressure and rotating the thumbs to release muscular tension. Work up and down the spine two or three times.

4 Move round so your partner can rest their head on your thighs, and with long, effleurage strokes, massage the length of the back from the neck right down to the buttocks and back up the sides of the trunk. Repeat three times.

5 Starting at the lower back, gently stroke up either side of the spine, making light feathery strokes with your fingertips. Repeat three times, making the strokes lighter each time, until they can barely be felt.

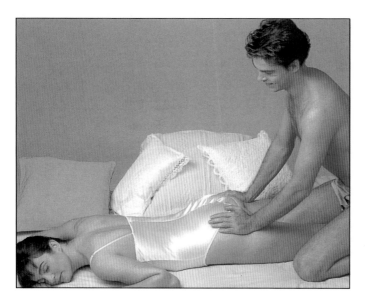

6 Left: Massage the lower back with some kneading. Using the flat, and in particular the heel, of the hand, knead the buttocks, then come back to the start and work over a different area. The nerves that cross this area relate to the man's groin, and the woman's uterus. The buttocks themselves are highly erogenous areas.

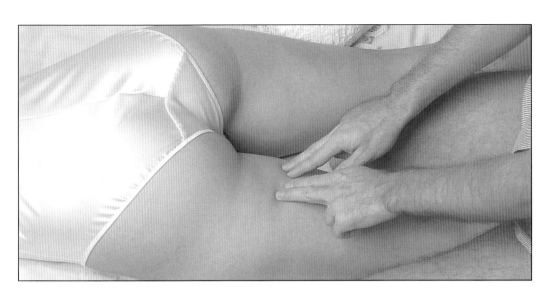

7 Curling your third and fourth fingers under, place your hands toward the top of the upper legs and circle your first and second fingers outward, one hand alternating with the other. This should be a slow, leisurely stroke with varying pressure.

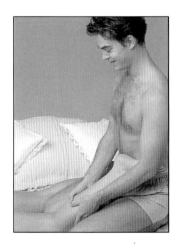

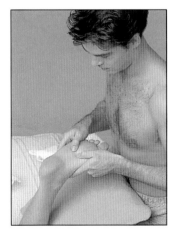

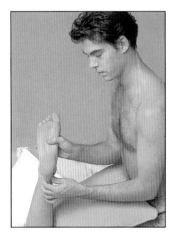

8 Support your partner's leg across your thigh and circle your thumbs over the calf, alternating the thumbs and applying firm pressure.

9 Raise your partner's foot, supporting its weight in your hands. Knead the instep firmly, using the thumbs to apply the pressure. Work all over the ball of the foot up toward the big toe.

10 Support your partner's foot in one hand, and place the thumb of that hand firmly over centre of the instep. This has a wonderful, calming effect. With the thumb and first finger of the other hand, stroke round the ankle using circular movements.

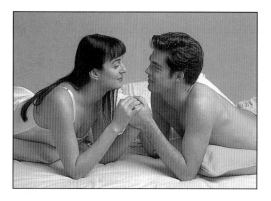

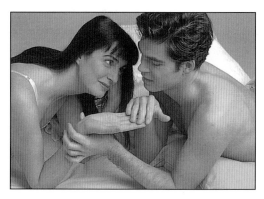

11 *At this stage, lie down facing each other, making sure you are both comfortable and well supported with plenty of cushions. Gently caress your partner's hands.*

12 *Gently stretch and release your partner's wrists, by flexing the hand backward and forwards. Softly stroke the inside of the palm with your fingers. Repeat on the other hand.*

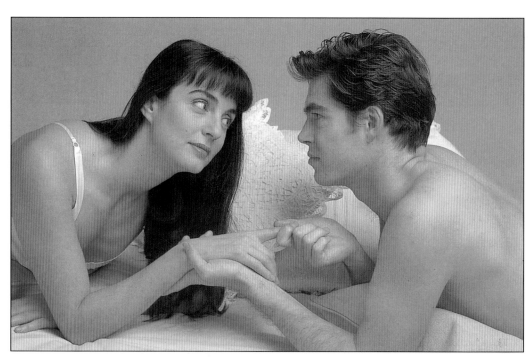

13 *Gently massage each finger, beginning with the thumb or little finger and working from the base joint to the tip. Try squeezing, rubbing and circular movements, and gentle pulling.*

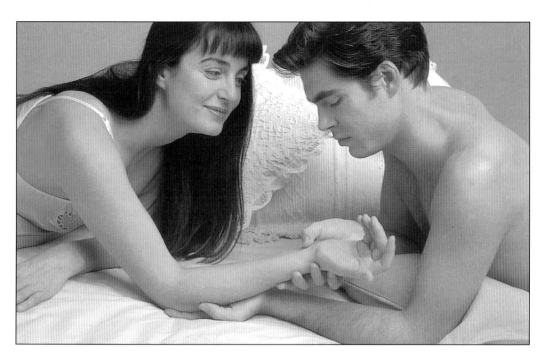

14 *Supporting your partner's elbow in one hand, use the other to caress and stroke the inside of the wrist just below the thumb, which is a particularly sensitive area. Continue working over the whole of the wrist area, using gentle circular thumb movements. Repeat on the other wrist.*

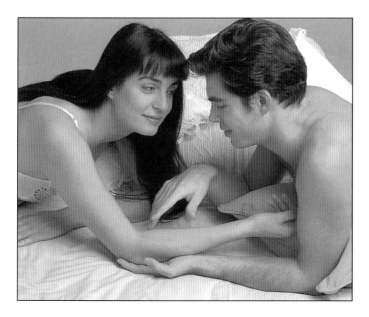

15 *Left: With feather strokes, use your fingers to stroke up the soft inner arm. This is a highly sensitive area when lightly touched and the effect is both stimulating and relaxing. Repeat on the other arm.*

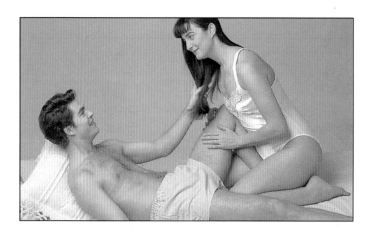

16 *Left: Use long* effleurage *strokes up and down the inner thigh area. Then massage closer to the highly erogenous region of the groin.*

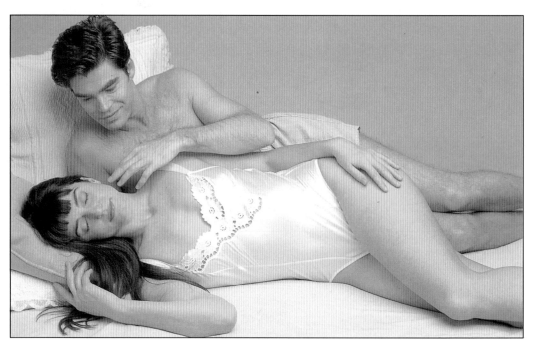

17 With a feathery touch, stroke across the shoulders and up the neck, covering the sides, front and back. You can run your fingers up through the hair as well. Spend more time caressing the base of the neck, which arouses strong, sexual responses.

18 *Right: Finally, trace round the ear with your fingers, starting at the outside and circling toward the centre. Continue with soft pinching movements round the outside edge and on the lobe, where you will be triggering sexual responses from the adrenal gland and sexual organs.*

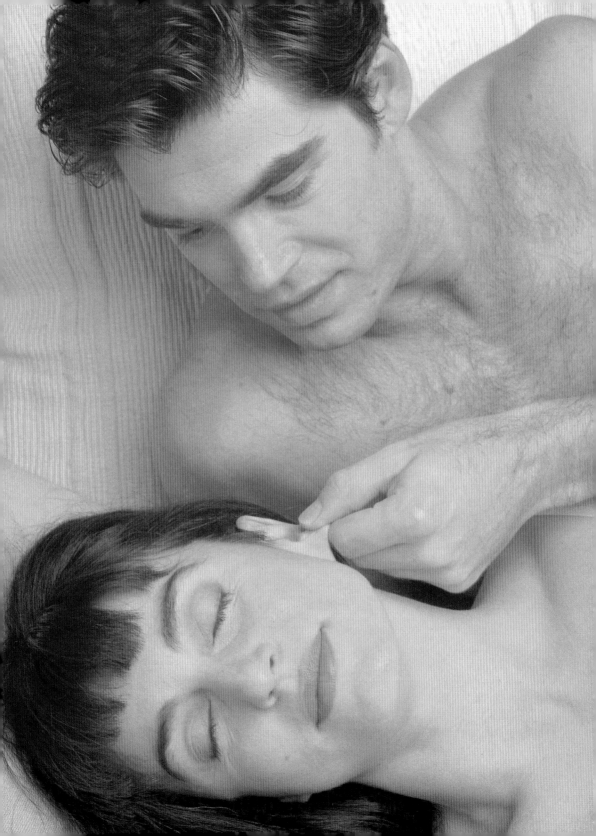

INSTANT MASSAGE

Sometimes, the idea of having tension in your shoulders and neck massaged away, without stopping to find the right place and the time to undress, is a particularly tempting one. There is increasing interest in learning how to do a shoulder massage with the minimum of disruption, especially in offices. Even at home, there are times when nothing is better than someone giving you a ten-minute shoulder and neck massage, in the comfort of an upright chair. There is no need to use oil if you prefer not to, and you can work through light clothing if simpler.

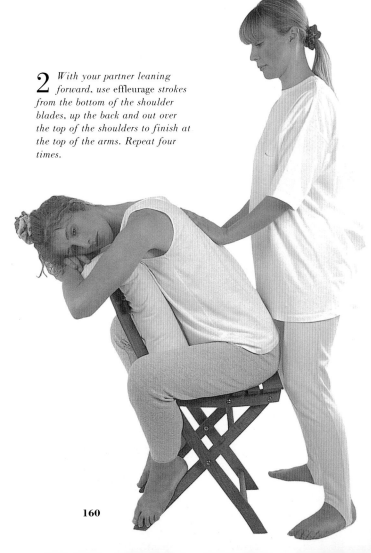

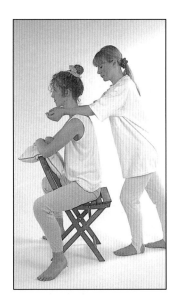

2 With your partner leaning forward, use effleurage strokes from the bottom of the shoulder blades, up the back and out over the top of the shoulders to finish at the top of the arms. Repeat four times.

1 Ask your partner to sit astride a chair facing the back. You can offer a folded towel or cushion for comfort. Standing behind your partner, begin by leaning on your forearms so that your weight presses down gently on to the fleshy part of the shoulders.

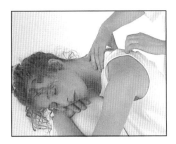 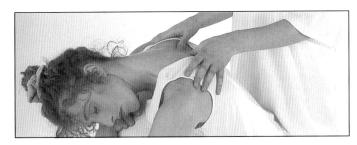

3 *With a firm* petrissage, *use both hands to knead out along the shoulders from the sides of the neck to the upper arms.*

4 *Starting as far down the lower back as you can, work up the spine with small circular frictions. Continue up the sides of the neck to* the base of the skull, then glide back down and work up again, this time moving out over the shoulders as you reach the top.

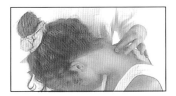 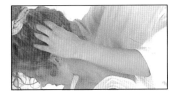 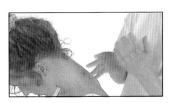

5 *Moving round to the side of the chair, tilt your partner's head forward and support it with one hand. With the thumb and finger of the bther hand, grasp the neck firmly and massage with circular movements, working up the neck and into the base of the skull.*

6 *Working from behind your partner again, massage the back of the head with both hands coming over the forehead and down to the temples with small circular pressures, moving the scalp against the skull. Lighten your touch at the temples.*

7 *First on one side and then the other, do some hacking across the fleshy parts of the shoulders and upper back, using the outer side of your hands to make short, brisk movements. Keep the wrists and hands very relaxed.*

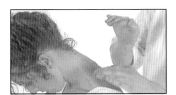 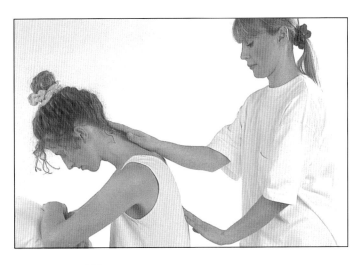

8 *Continue with a brisk cupping action across each shoulder, working on one side at a time.*

9 *Right: Finish the sequence by gently stroking down the entire back with one hand following the other. Repeat five times with each stroke getting lighter.*

REFLEXOLOGY

Most people enjoy massage to the feet – one of the most sensitive parts of the body. All foot massage is beneficial and relaxing, but reflexology provides a more specific method of working to diagnose problems and stimulate health in the whole body. It is based on the principle that the body can be divided into ten vertical zones, each corresponding to an area of the foot, so that the feet are in effect a map of the body. A sensitive area of the foot indicates a problem in the corresponding organ of the body and by working on the appropriate trouble-spot, the larger problem can be helped. Reflexology can be an effective way of relieving pain and helping to restore the body's natural balance and well-being.

FOOT CHARTS

The foot charts are only guidelines for interpretation. When you find a tender or congested part of the foot you may look for that part on the charts and see approximately which reflex the tenderness lies on. This is only a rough guide because every pair of feet are different and will not be the same shape as your chart. Also, the charts are two-dimensional and your body is three-dimensional and therefore the reflexes on your feet reflect this. In reality your organs overlap each other, whereas the charts are much simplified for clarity, to give an idea of where things are.

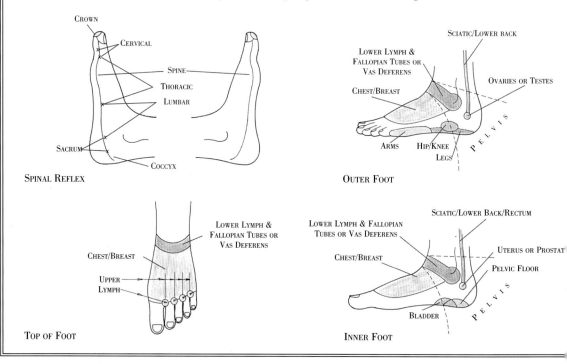

THE BACKGROUND

The concept of using the body's reflexes for therapeutic purposes is not new – the early Chinese developed the technique of acupressure thousands of years ago. This provided the basis of knowledge about reflex zones and points and connections between different parts of the body. We know that the early Chinese, Japanese, Indians and Egyptians worked on the feet to promote good health, and many of the long-established principles developed by these civilizations are used in modern-day practice.

Reflexology as it is known today is based largely on the work of Dr William Fitzgerald and Eunice Ingham. Dr Fitzgerald devised his own system of acupressure points which produced an analgesic effect when stimulated. He found that the body could be divided into ten zones running from the top of the head to the tips of the toes, and that everything occuring in a specific zone of the body could affect the organs and other parts of the body in that zone. The theory was refined in the 1930s by a young physiotherapist called Eunice Ingham, who introduced a special grip technique and the action of the thumb on the foot and developed a more intricate zone system. Since then, the system has been further refined into the internationally recognized method that is practiced today.

Modern reflexology offers tremendous health benefits: it reduces stress, improves circulation, cleanses the body of impurities and toxins, and can revitalize energy levels.

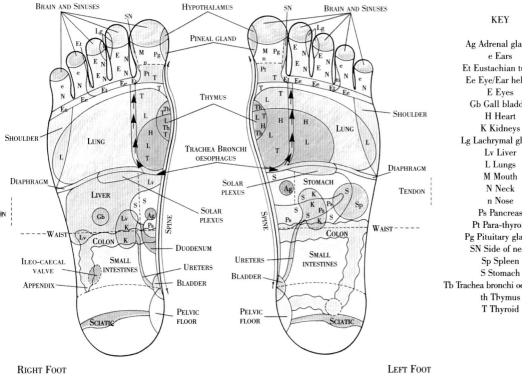

KEY

Ag Adrenal glands
e Ears
Et Eustachian tubes
Ee Eye/Ear helper
E Eyes
Gb Gall bladder
H Heart
K Kidneys
Lg Lachrymal glands
Lv Liver
L Lungs
M Mouth
N Neck
n Nose
Ps Pancreas
Pt Para-thyroid
Pg Pituitary glands
SN Side of neck
Sp Spleen
S Stomach
Tb Trachea bronchi oesophagus
th Thymus
T Thyroid

RIGHT FOOT

LEFT FOOT

BASIC REFLEXOLOGY TECHNIQUES

THE TREATMENT

Advanced diagnosis is a trained professional skill but some basic techniques can easily be used in a foot massage. You can also use them to work on your own feet, sitting with one ankle supported on the opposite thigh.

The following points will ensure a relaxing session:

● Work with your partner's foot in your lap or supported at the right height with cushions or bolsters.

● Your partner can sit in a comfortable chair with a footstool or small table to raise the feet.

● Ensure the back, neck and knees are properly supported, so your partner can relax completely.

● The massage is given without oil. You can dust the feet with talcum powder or work directly on the skin, if you prefer.

● Make sure your nails are short and well filed.

The following sequence of movements offers an introduction to reflexology. It is necessary to hold the foot correctly so that all points can be reached and stimulated with ease. The hands will swap their holding and working roles according to the part of the foot to be reached, so practice with both hands.

Apart from proper holding, the main principle to observe is leverage. Use the rest of the fingers in opposition to the working thumb to obtain more effective contact with the foot, or the thumb in opposition to the working finger in finger walking.

GREETING THE FEET

Below: The initial contact with the feet sets the tone for the whole treatment. Gently holding both feet relaxes them, allows you to learn about your partner and establishes a relationship.

ANKLE ROTATION

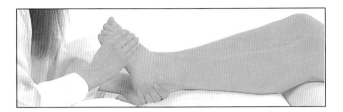

Begin with some relaxing movements. Stabilize the ankle by holding the right foot in the left hand, supporting the heel.

Gently wrap the fingers of the working hand below the base of the toes. Rotate the foot several times in each direction.

ANKLE STRETCH

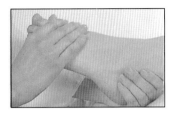

Using the same hold as for the ankle rotation, stretch the foot back and forth slowly to release tension in the Achilles tendon, taking care not to force the ankle joint. Then work all round the ankle, applying pressure. This area corresponds to the reproductive organs, legs and lower back.

SOLAR PLEXUS RELAXATION

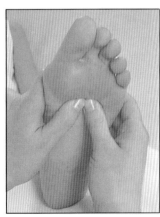

Place both thumbs on the solar plexus point located in the centre of the ball of the foot where there is a little indentation. This is a good relaxation exercise, particularly if your partner is very tense or nervous. You can also work on both feet simultaneously.

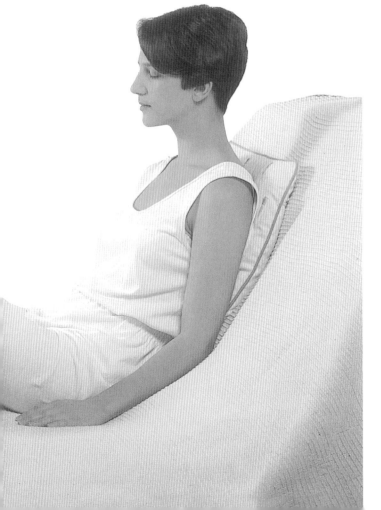

THUMB HOOKING

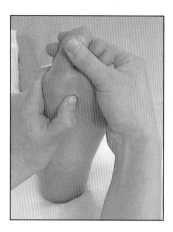

Place the outer corner of the thumb on a reflex point, with the thumb flat. Bend the thumb at the first joint to apply pressure, and pull back across the point. Use the other fingers for counter-pressure and raise the wrist to increase the pressure. Hooking is used to stimulate points that are too small for the walking technique (see right), such as the pituitary point, the solar plexus and lymph drainage points, and any point of soreness.

THUMB WALKING

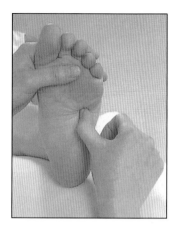

This is the principal technique for covering large areas. Thumb walking starts in the same way as the thumb hook and then the outside corner of the flexed thumb is rocked slightly forward. Maintain steady pressure as the thumb walks, avoiding an "on-off" movement. Press along the diaphragm line under the ball of the foot, then stimulate the spinal area along the main arch of foot from the heel to the big toe.

FINGER WALKING

1,2 This technique is used to work on the top of the feet. The principle is the same as for thumb walking: flexing the first finger joint and rocking forward. With the holding hand, support and spread the toes, and push on the ball of the foot with the thumb of the working hand to provide leverage. Finger walk from the base of the little toe up to the ankle. Begin again, walking between the troughs of the next toes, toward the inside of the foot.

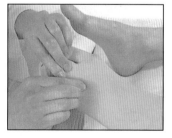 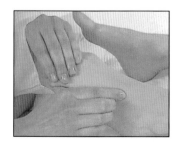

This helps to relieve tension in the chest and lung area, and the areas for lymph drainage and vocal chords which are located between the big toe and second toe at the top of the foot.

STROKING THE FEET

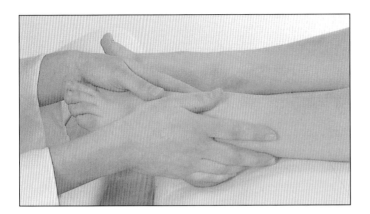

Left: Using alternate hands, stroke the foot softly from the ankles to the toes to smooth and relax the whole area of each foot.

DESSERT STROKE

Right: Take the foot in both hands and slide the hands gently up and down. Dessert strokes are enjoyable and can be used throughout the treatment to soothe and relax your partner after a sensitive reflex has been worked on. Always end the session with dessert strokes to rebalance the whole foot.

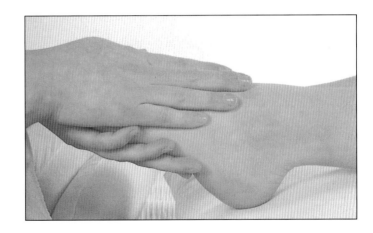

For an effective treatment:

● Explore the foot with the outside edge of the thumb, by the nail, but be careful not to dig with your nail.
● Make regular eye contact with your partner to check responses to specific pressures and to detect painful or sensitive areas.

● Pay extra attention to sensitive areas, which may feel granular, as these are usually due to calcification or deposits of lymph fluid. Work on them thoroughly to disperse the blockages and release energy in the zone.
● Work on each area of the foot several times and make sure that no area is left out.

● Work through each foot once to find sensitive areas and then a second time to reintegrate the foot and body.
● Join the movements and areas of the foot with dessert strokes.
● Always keep contact with at least one hand.
● Knuckling can be used to cover large areas of the foot.

USEFUL ADDRESSES

MASSAGE

ORGANIZATIONS

Association of Physical and Natural Therapists
93 Parkhurst Road
Horley
Surrey RH6 8EX
Tel: 0293 775467

British Massage Therapy Council
9 Elm Road
Worthing
Sussex BN11 1PG

Institute for Complementary Medicine
Unit 4
Tavern Quay
London SE16
Tel: 071-237 5165

PRACTITIONERS AND COURSES

The Bluestone Clinic
34 Devonshire Place
London W1N 1PE
Tel: 071-935 7933

Champneys
Chesham Road
Wiggington
Tring
Herts HP23 6HY
Tel: 0442 863351

Henlow Grange
Henlow
Bedfordshire SG16 6BD
Tel: 0462 811111

Grayshott Hall
Headley Road
Grayshott
Nr Hindhead
Surrey GU26 6JJ
Tel: 0428 604331

London College of Massage
5 Newman Passage
London W1P 3PF
Tel: 071-323 3574

London School of Sports Massage
88 Cambridge Street
London SW1V 4QG
Tel: 071-233 5962

Massage Training Institute
24 Highbury Grove
London N5 2EA
Tel: 071-226 5313

Northern Institute of Massage
100 Waterloo Road
Blackpool FY4 1AW

American Massage Therapy Association
820 Davies Street
Evanston
IL 60201
USA

Boulder School of Massage Therapy
PO Box 4573
Boulder
CO 80306
USA

The Connecticut Center for Massage Therapy
75 Kitts Lane
Newington
CT 06111
USA

Australian Natural Therapists Association
PO Box 522
Sutherland
NSW 2232
Australia

South African Institute of Health and Beauty Therapists
PO Box 56318
Pinegowrie
22123
Johannesburg
South Africa

REFLEXOLOGY

The British School of Reflexology
92 Sheering Road
Old Harlow
Essex CN17 0JW
Tel: 0279 429060

British School of Reflex Zone Therapy
87 Oakington Avenue
Wembley Park
London HA9 8HY
Tel: 081-908 2201

International Institute of Reflexology
15 Hartfield Close
Tonbridge
Kent TN10 4JP

Reflexologists' Society
39 Presbury Road
Cheltenham
Glos GL52 2PT
Tel: 0242 512601

International Institute of Reflexology
PO Box 12642
5650 First Avenue North
St Petersburg
FLA 33733-2642
USA

FURTHER READING

MASSAGE

Nigel Dawes and Fiona Harrold, *Massage Cures*, Thorsons 1990

George Downing, *The Massage Book*, Wildwood House, 1973

Fiona Harrold, *The Massage Manual*, Headline, 1992

Tina Heinl, *Baby Massage*, Prentice Hall, 1983

Nitya Lacroix, *Massage for Total Relaxation*, Dorling Kindersley, 1991

Sensual Massage, Dorling Kindersley, 1989

Lucinda Lidell, *The Massage Book*, Ebury Press, 1984

Clare Maxwell-Hudson, *The Complete Book of Massage*, Dorling Kindersley, 1988

Sara Thomas, *Massage for Common Ailments*, Sidgwick & Jackson, 1989

Jacqueline Young, *Self Massage*, Thorsons, 1992

REFLEXOLOGY

Dwight C. Byers, *Better Health with Foot Reflexology*, Ingham Publishing Inc., 1983

Kevin and Barbara Kunz, *The Complete Guide to Foot Reflexology*, Prentice Hall, 1982

Laura Norman with Thomas Cowan, *The Reflexology Handbook*, Judy Piatkus, 1988

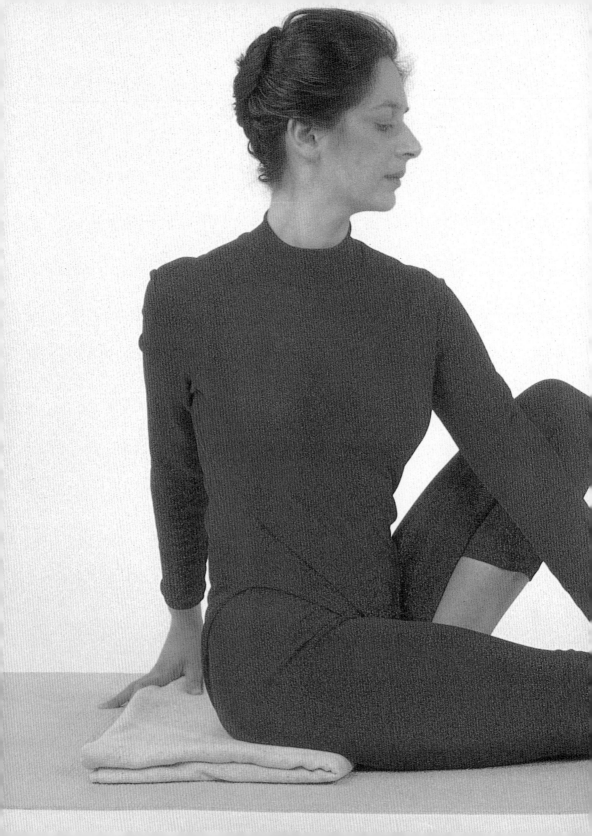

YOGA

THE IYENGAR BASICS

A powerful antidote to the stresses of modern-day life, yoga is a practical philosophy that aims at uniting the body, mind and spirit for health and fulfilment. A fit and supple body can be developed through the practice of postures (asanas). These easy-to-follow exercises, especially chosen for beginners, work on all the bodily systems, toning the muscles, stimulating the circulation and improving overall health. The benefits are not merely physical: as the postures are mastered and techniques introduced for relaxation and breath control, you will find that yoga has the power to calm the mind, increase your concentration and give the ability to cope with tension. It is a complete system for personal development, promoting total physical and spiritual well-being.

The authors wish to acknowledge their indebtedness to Yogacharya Sri B.K.S. Iyengar for his help and support in the preparation of this work.

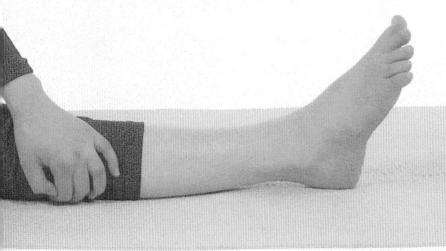

THE GIFT OF YOGA

Yoga is one of India's wonderful gifts to mankind. One of its valuable qualities is that it builds up a store of physical health through the practice of a system of exercises called asanas which keep the body cleansed and fit. Yoga believes that exercise is essential for speedy removal of toxins and for keeping blood circulation and all internal processes functioning smoothly.

Having dealt with the physical side of life, yoga turns to the mental. Here different breathing exercises or techniques quieten the mind and brain, offering inner peace and an ability to face upheavals and deal with problems.

Uniting both these aspects is the philosophy of yoga which has stood the test of time, bidding humanity to review its thinking and its conduct, and to turn away from violence, dishonesty and greed – a review of life much needed in the present day.

Yoga therefore has a role both in everyday practical life, and in the more thoughtful, idealistic scheme of things. Its value needs to be experienced and savoured.

YOGA – A BRIEF OVERVIEW

Yoga has been practised in India for over two millenia. Stories and legends from ancient times all testify to the existence of yoga, and to the practitioners and divinities associated with it.

Indian literature is a storehouse of knowledge about yoga covering every conceivable level. Roughly in chronological order are the *Vedas* (books of scriptural knowledge), the *Upanisads* (philosophical speculations), and their commentaries; then the *Puranas* (ancient cosmologies), and the two epics, the *Ramayana* and the *Mahabharata*. The *Mahabharata* contains within itself that masterpiece of Indian scripture, the *Bhagavad Gita*. Toward the end of the Vedic period comes the aphoristic literature, with the "Yoga Aphorisms" of Patanjali of especial interest to yoga students. There are, besides, whole bodies of works both ancient (pre-Christian) and more modern dealing with various aspects of yoga and yoga philosophy, testifying to the continued relevance of yoga as a discipline.

Yoga is considered to be a philosophy, a science and an art. It has eight clearly defined aspects and, in its purest form, is a complete system capable of answering all human needs. However, it has always been, and still is, used as a basis for other activities and disciplines. Today, for example, physiotherapy and exercise classes often adapt movements from yoga postures.

Different schools of yoga through the ages have

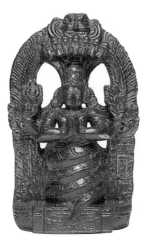

Patanjali is the legendary founder of yoga. According to tradition he brought to humanity serenity of spirit through the philosophy of yoga, clarity of speech by his work on grammar, and health of body by his work on medicine.

Indian iconography gives him a half human, half serpent form, as depicted in this modern sculpture.

stressed different aspects, but all branches have a common ideological basis, of seeking the betterment of individual yoga practitioners, and, in a broader context, of humanity.

The word yoga comes from the Sanskrit root *"yuj"* meaning to join or yoke, implying the integration (or joining) of every aspect of a human being from the innermost to the external. Another frequently used definition of yoga is that of union of the individual spirit with the universal, since that is its highest aim.

As a philosophy, yoga is unusual in that it insists that the practice of postures – apparently physical exercises – and breathing techniques is essential in order to lead a worthy and satisfying life. A whole doctrine attaches to the postural and breathing aspects of yoga. The parallel classical Western concept of *"mens sana in corpore sano"* – a healthy body in a healthy mind – has always been recognized and is finding increasing emphasis today.

PATANJALI AND THE YOGA SUTRAS

The first semi-historical, semi-mythological figure in yoga is that of the sage Patanjali who lived some time in the pre-Christian era – one estimate suggests about 220 BC. He is traditionally said to be the author of works on medicine, grammar and yoga. Together these cover the fields of the body, the intellect and the spirit. His treatise on yoga is called the "Yoga Sutras" or "Yoga Aphorisms" and it is still considered authoritative today.

The *Yoga Sutras* summarizes all the various aspects of yoga and systematizes them. According to Patanjali, yoga consists of eight limbs, which are all equally important and are related as parts of a whole. They are as follows:

1. Five universal commandments (*yama*) aimed at creating a "better" world: not harming anyone or anything; truthfulness; non-stealing; leading a godly, chaste life; and being non-grasping.

2. Five personal disciplines (*niyama*): cleanliness; contentedness; self-discipline; self-study and study of the scriptures; and dedication to God.

3. Practice of postures (*asana*): devoted and conscientious practice of the various types of posture.

4. Practice of breath control (*pranayama*): practising breathing techniques with care and discrimination.

5. Detachment from worldly activities (*pratyahara*): developing a non-attached attitude of body and mind.

6. Concentration (*dharana*): Being able to hold on to a subject mentally.

7. Meditation (*dhyana*): developing a quiet, meditative state.

8. Trance or a state of bliss (*samadhi*): reaching a state of absorption in a subject or in the Divine.

THE INFLUENCE OF B.K.S. IYENGAR

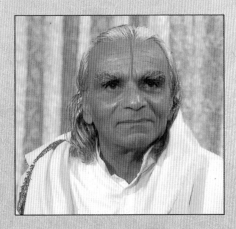

he work of B.K.S. Iyengar confirms him as a modern pioneer of yoga. He has explained and exemplified all the traditional aspects of the subject as laid down by Patanjali. He has rediscovered and systematized a whole range of postures and breathing techniques, making them accessible to yoga practitioners of all levels, throughout the world.

Most importantly, B.K.S. Iyengar has worked extensively on the therapeutic effects of yoga. His authority is acknowledged throughout the world by all schools of yoga and his books *Light on Yoga* and *Light on Pranayama* are modern classics. He has received numerous titles and awards for his services to yoga from the Government of India and from various educational organizations.

The postures and breath control techniques given in this book are based on B.K.S. Iyengar's work.

TOWARD PHYSICAL WELLBEING

Yoga is an ineffable art which, though backed by a very logical philosophy, does not reveal itself by theorization. Only by practice does one experience the effects of the various asanas and pranayamas on the body, mind and spirit.

Why the body becomes supple and efficient through yoga can easily be understood. Why and how yoga affects the mind is not so immediately apparent. But why it should affect the spirit – will-power, feeling of well-being, energy – seems to defy all logic.

On reading this you may think, "This is all very interesting, but it is not for me". However, if you practise some of the postures in the way they have been described, you are likely to be agreeably surprised. Although you may find that the postures are more difficult than they look, and not all your joints may be working as well as you expected, do not give up. The postures will soon begin to help you with any physical weaknesses you may have. They will also stretch your mind and enhance your concentration.

SCOPE OF THE COURSE

The aim of this course is to provide a basic introduction to the theory and practice of yoga. The major part, *Toward Physical Wellbeing*, deals with 41 postures and variants – the Asanas – which may be attempted by beginners of all ages. Principal techniques are given with clear illustrations and stages so that the postures may be easily followed by everyone.

A ten-week course is included to guide your practice systematically and progressively. Daily practice is suggested, but if you cannot do this the course will take longer. A few necessary precautions are given to make sure your practice will be safe. Some general practice points are also given.

In addition, there is a section giving postures which are helpful for some common problems – headaches, stiffness and pain in the neck and shoulders, backache and stiffness of the hips. There is also a programme of postures suitable to be done during menstruation.

In *Toward Mental Peace*,

guidance is given in some simple relaxation and breathing techniques to show how these calm the mind.

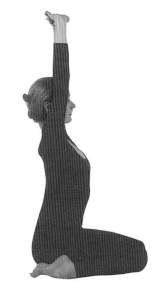

HOME PRACTICE

There are several ways of planning practice at home. These depend on a number of factors such as time available, family and other duties, and individual requirements.

Time

There are no set rules about when to practise, or how long. Clearly the more yoga is done, the greater the benefit.

Some people prefer to practise in the morning, others in the evening. It is also possible to break up practice sessions so that they slot in in shorter periods whenever is convenient during the day – even if only for 10 minutes at a time.

Family and other Duties

Practice may be modified according to circumstances. At times it may need to be geared to fulfilling family and other obligations effectively. In this case it is important to plan the time and programme for practice carefully so as to derive maximum benefit. For example, if you have only 10 or 20 minutes to spare and are being faced with a heavy workload or stressful situation, supported Sarvangasana (nos. 37 and 38) and Setu Bandha Sarvangasana (no. 39) or Viparita Karani (no. 40) may be the most appropriate.

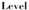

Level

The practice of postures and pranayama will vary according to the level and experience of the student. The basic poses should be practised on a regular basis and should never be forgotten. One method is to vary the type of postures done each day, for instance, standing poses one day and sitting poses the next. Always include inverted poses. Beginners should concentrate more on standing poses.

Individual Needs

In home practice you have to be sensitive to your own needs and to be aware which postures are helpful in different circumstances. For example, standing poses are invigorating, whereas forward bends are calming.

This is one approach to practice. The other is to discipline yourself to do a particular programme irrespective of personal inclination. The first approach makes you sensitive and the second develops will-power. Both need to be learnt.

Where there is a health problem for which a certain group of postures are prescribed, then this particular programme should be adhered to.

Structure

Yoga practice should have a structure. A basic guide is to start with simple poses or those which allow the body to stretch; then to continue with the main group or groups of poses selected for that day, and to end with relaxing poses that allow the work done to be assimilated by the body.

Self-discipline

Practising at home requires and develops self-discipline and an independent understanding of the postures. It is a good idea to begin by remembering some of the postures and instructions given. The building up of correct habits will give a firm foundation in yoga, leading to confidence in practice and greater knowledge.

Repetition of Postures

It is usual to repeat some of the postures when practising, such as standing poses, sitting poses and twists, so long as this does not cause fatigue. However, do not repeat the inverted postures and recuperative positions.

Timings in the Postures

Guidance is given in the Asana section for the timing of each posture. In the beginning do not stay long in the postures, until they become familiar and you gain stamina. Do not strain to hold a posture. Gradually increase the time spent in each so that the postures – as well as your health – improve.

Breathing in the Postures

Do upward movements with an inhalation, downward movements with an exhalation. That is, start a movement at the beginning of an inhalation or exhalation, and conclude it at the end of the same breath if possible. Do not hold the breath in the postures.

Menstruation

Women should not do inverted poses during menstruation as these interfere with the natural outflow of blood. There is a whole range of postures which are suitable at this time – see Asanas for Menstruation.

CAUTION

This course is not intended for those suffering from the following conditions:

- cancer or benign tumours
- detached retina
- diabetes
- epilepsy including petit mal
- heart disease
- high blood pressure
- HIV
- Meniere's disease
- Multiple Sclerosis (MS)
- Myalgic Encephalomyelitis (ME)
- physical handicaps
- pregnancy
- recent post-operative conditions

In such cases, please seek the advice of an experienced teacher.

THE ASANAS

There are many different types of yoga postures – Indian texts sometimes mention 840,000! – but in practice only about 20 or 30 principal ones were in regular use until recently. However, through the work of B.K.S. Iyengar, over 200 postures are now being practised by yoga students all over the world. The system of postures has come to be accepted as a subject in its own right, since great attention is paid to the precision and correct execution of the movements.

The postures (asanas) are all anatomically and physiologically sound. They are a guide to the variety of movement attainable by the human body. In the Iyengar method they have been categorized according to level of difficulty, to be practised by those from beginner level to advanced stages.

The postures are grouped according to the positioning of the body – standing, sitting, twisting, prone, supine, inverted and balancing. They incorporate slow and quick motion and teach concentration, dynamism and stillness. They have important therapeutic effects, since the entire organic structure is invigorated and toned by practice of the postures. Muscle tone is automatically improved. The yoga student will benefit from increasing health, stamina and agility.

At the psychological level, the postures have their own intrinsic value since they are challenging and interesting to do. They also have a direct balancing effect on certain psychological disorders – thus, they can "liven up" a lethargic and depressed person, or calm a frenetic, distressed person.

BEFORE YOU BEGIN

There are some basic guidelines which should be followed before beginning yoga practice:

● Wait for 4–5 hours after a heavy meal or 2–3 hours after a light snack.

● Empty the bladder and move the bowels before you start. Supported Sarvangasana (no. 38) and Ardha Halasana (no. 36) will help.

● Practise in loose-fitting clothing and bare feet.

● Work on a non-slip mat or floor. Especially in the winter, the floor should not be too cold.

● Fold blankets neatly when preparing to use them, as any creases will disturb your practice.

● Remove hard contact lenses.

● Seek advice if you experience difficulties in practice. Your difficulty may be a common one, and there is likely to be a solution. In the meantime, avoid straining.

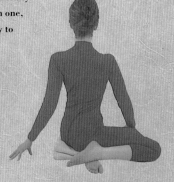

STANDING POSES

1 · TADASANA
MOUNTAIN POSE

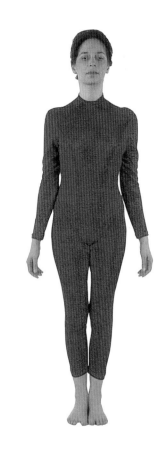

*This is the first posture to be learnt. It is the basic standing pose,
with which they start and finish.*

*Although Tadasana is practised from the beginning, it is difficult to master
as it involves bringing the energies of the body and mind into equilibrium in
a static pose. This can only be done when postural defects have been
corrected by working on a variety of asanas. For this reason, beginners
should become familiar with the postures gradually.*

*Stand with the feet together, and
big toes, heels and ankle bones
touching. Keep the knees straight
and pull up the thigh muscles.
Stretch the legs up, extend the spine
and lift the front of the body. Take
the shoulders back, shoulder blades
in and allow the arms to hang
loosely at the sides of the trunk.
Relax the hands and keep the
palms facing the hips. Extend the
neck up and relax the face. Look
straight ahead. Concentrate on
centering the body: balance the
weight evenly on both feet; create
awareness in the soles of the feet
and stretch them equally. Be
conscious of extending the right
and left sides of the body evenly.
Keep the chest open.*

   *Stay in the posture for 30–60
seconds when practising Tadasana
on its own; less when doing it as a
stage of other poses.*

NOTES ON THE POSTURES

Read the following notes regarding
individual groups of postures
before beginning practice.

Standing poses
● Do not jump into the postures if
you have a bad back or injured
knees.
● Do not strain the knees when
straightening them.
● Do not hold the breath.
● Do not strain the throat or the
abdomen.

Sitting poses
● Sit on one or two folded
blankets in order not to strain the
lower back. Reduce the height
when you are more flexible.
● Do not use force to straighten
the legs but extend them
carefully.

Twists
● Sit on folded blankets to raise
the base of the spine. You will
then be able to turn the whole
trunk.
● Do not tense the abdomen.

Inverted poses
● Avoid these postures during
menstruation. Postures to be done
at this time are given in the section
– "Asanas for Menstruation".
● These poses should feel
comfortable. If you experience
pressure in any part of the head or
neck, your blankets may need
adjusting, or you may have gone
up awkwardly.
● Seek advice if you have or have
had any head or neck injuries, or
any medical condition affecting
the eyes, ears or brain.

2 · VRKSASANA
TREE POSE

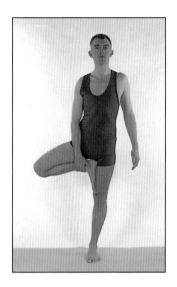

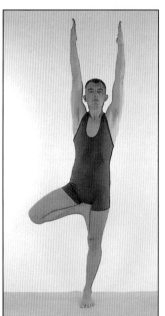

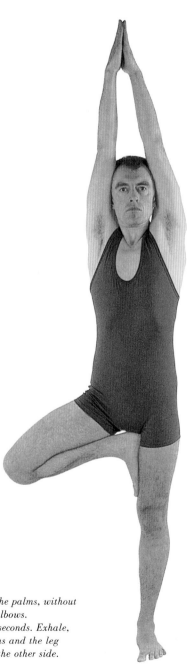

1 *Stand in Tadasana (no. 1).*
Without disturbing the left
leg, bend the right leg to the side.
Catch the ankle and place the foot
at the top of the inner left thigh.
Take it as high as possible. Press
the right knee back, in line with
the right hip.

2 *Inhale and take the arms over*
the head with the palms
facing each other. Straighten the
elbows and stretch the arms and
trunk up. Stand firmly on the left
foot so that you do not overbalance.
Stretch the leg up.

3 *Right: Join the palms, without*
bending the elbows.
  Stay for 20–30 seconds. Exhale,
then bring the arms and the leg
down. Repeat on the other side.

3 · UTTHITA TRIKONASANA
EXTENDED TRIANGLE POSE

Trikonasana is one of the most important standing poses. Learn the various points gradually, incorporate them into your practice and build on them.

● *If you have a bad back or injured knees, do not jump into standing poses.*

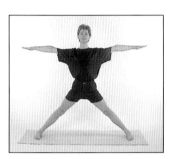

1 Stand in Tadasana (no. 1). With a deep inhalation, jump the feet about 3½–4 ft (105–120 cm) apart, at the same time raising the arms to shoulder level, palms face down. Line up the feet to be level and facing forward.

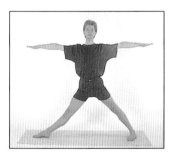

2 Turn the left foot about 15° in and the right foot about 90° out. Line up the right heel to be exactly opposite the left instep. As you turn the left foot in, rotate the left leg outwards. As you turn the right foot out, rotate the whole leg in the same direction (that is, to the right). Keep the knees tight and lift the trunk.

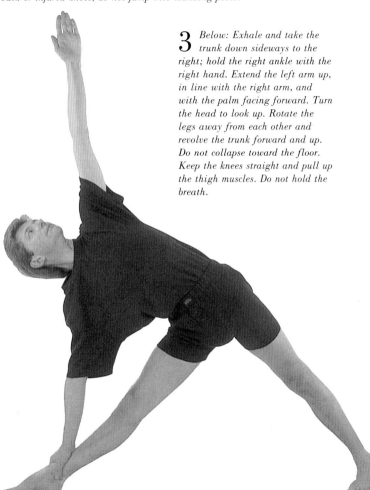

3 Below: Exhale and take the trunk down sideways to the right; hold the right ankle with the right hand. Extend the left arm up, in line with the right arm, and with the palm facing forward. Turn the head to look up. Rotate the legs away from each other and revolve the trunk forward and up. Do not collapse toward the floor. Keep the knees straight and pull up the thigh muscles. Do not hold the breath.

Stay for 20–30 seconds. Inhale and come up to 2. Turn the feet to the centre. Rest the arms for a moment so that you do not feel fatigue (you may place them on the hips). Line up the feet again. Repeat on the other side. Come up, then exhale, jump the feet together and bring the arms down.

4 · UTTHITA PARSVAKONASANA
EXTENDED LATERAL ANGLE POSE

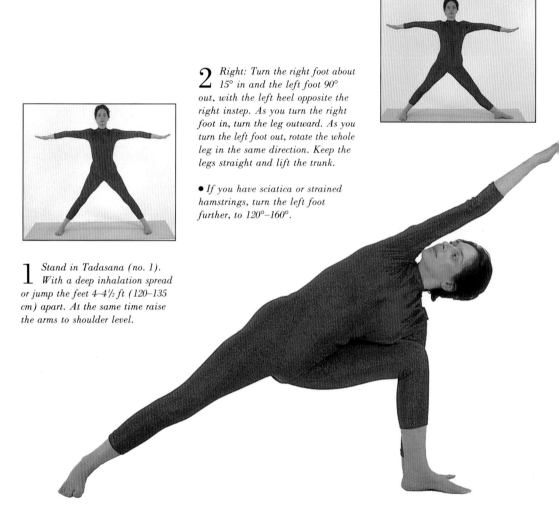

2 *Right: Turn the right foot about 15° in and the left foot 90° out, with the left heel opposite the right instep. As you turn the right foot in, turn the leg outward. As you turn the left foot out, rotate the whole leg in the same direction. Keep the legs straight and lift the trunk.*

• *If you have sciatica or strained hamstrings, turn the left foot further, to 120°–160°.*

1 *Stand in Tadasana (no. 1). With a deep inhalation spread or jump the feet 4–4½ ft (120–135 cm) apart. At the same time raise the arms to shoulder level.*

3 Keep the right leg firm and bend the left leg to 90°, with the shin perpendicular and the thigh parallel to the ground. Exhale and take the trunk sideways down to the left. Bend from the hips, not the waist. Place the left palm or fingertips on the floor by the outer edge of the left foot.

Turn the right arm and stretch it over the head, palm face down. Turn the head and look up. Keeping the right leg and both arms straight, revolve the whole trunk upward. Stretch the right side of the body toward the fingertips. Relax the face and breathe normally.

Stay for 20–30 seconds. Inhale

and come up. Turn the feet to the centre and rest the arms on the hips. Repeat on the other side. Come up to step 2, then exhale, and jump back to Tadasana.

• If breathing becomes strained, come up and rest, or face the ground till the breath returns to normal.

5 · VIRABHADRASANA I
WARRIOR POSE I

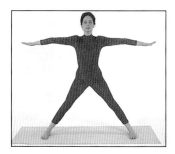

1 Stand in Tadasana (no. 1). With a deep inhalation, spread or jump the feet 4–4½ ft (120–135 cm) apart, raising the arms to shoulder level.

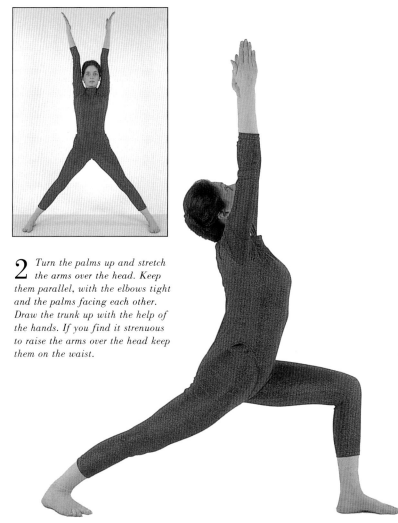

2 Turn the palms up and stretch the arms over the head. Keep them parallel, with the elbows tight and the palms facing each other. Draw the trunk up with the help of the hands. If you find it strenuous to raise the arms over the head keep them on the waist.

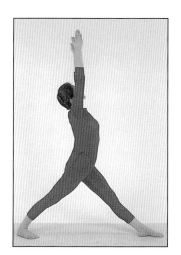

3 Turn the right leg and foot 45° in, and the left foot 90° out. At the same time turn the hips and trunk to the left. Make the left and right sides of the body parallel by bringing the right hip forward and taking the left hip slightly further back.

4 Exhale and bend the left leg to a right angle. Stretch the whole body up. Move the shoulder blades in and open the chest. Take the head back and look up. Do not strain the neck and throat. Keep the back leg firm and maintain the turn of the hips and trunk to the left. Stretch up to the maximum.

Stay for 20–30 seconds. Inhale and come up. Turn to the centre. Rest the arms and line up the feet. Repeat on the other side. Come up, then exhale and jump into Tadasana.

6. VIRABHADRASANA II
WARRIOR POSE II

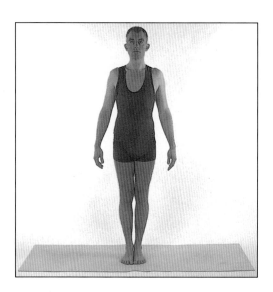

1 Stand in Tadasana (no. 1).

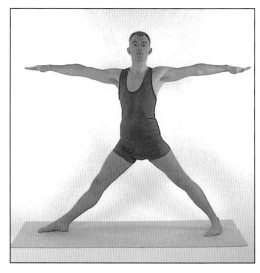

3 Turn the left foot about 15° in and the right foot 90° out. Line up the feet, with the right heel opposite the left instep. While turning the left foot in, rotate the left leg outward. While turning the right foot out, rotate the whole leg together with the foot. Keep both knees tight. Lift up the trunk from the hips.

● If you have sciatica, turn the right foot 120°–160°.

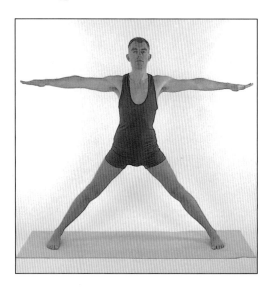

2 With a deep inhalation spread or jump the feet 4–4½ ft (120–135 cm) apart, raising the arms to shoulder level.

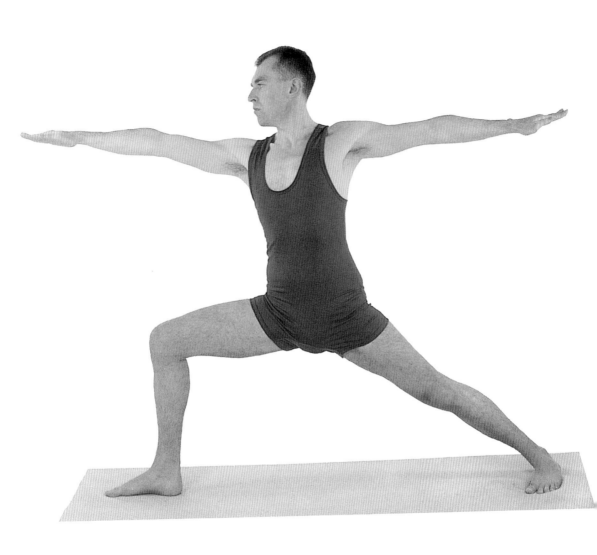

4 With an exhalation, bend the right leg to a right angle, keeping the left leg straight. Extend the trunk vertically up and stretch the arms horizontally to the sides, palms face down. Turn the head to the right. Pull the left arm slightly to the left so that the trunk does not lean to the right. Lift the chest. Relax the face and breathe normally.

Stay for 20–30 seconds. Inhale and come up. Turn the feet to the centre and line them up. Rest the arms if necessary.

Repeat on the other side. Come up, then exhale and jump into Tadasana.

7. PARSVOTTANASANA
EXTREME SIDEWAYS STRETCH

FULL POSE

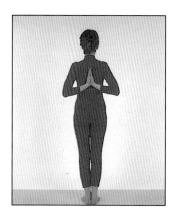 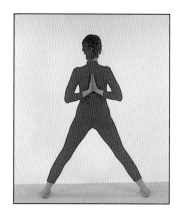 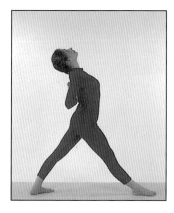

1 *Stand in Tadasana (no. 1). Join the palms behind the back in Namaste (for method, see box on facing page).*

2 *With a deep inhalation, jump the feet 3½– 4 ft (105–120 cm) apart. Line up the toes to make them level.*

3 *Turn the left leg and foot about 45° in, and the right foot 90° out. Turn the hips and trunk to the right. Stretch the trunk up and take the head back. Do not strain the throat.*

4 *Right: Exhale and bend down over the right leg. Keep both legs straight and make the hips level. Stretch down as far as you can, then relax the head.*

Stay for 20–30 seconds. Inhale and come up. Turn to the front, without releasing the hands. Line up the feet, then repeat on the other side.

Come up, turn to the front, then exhale and jump into Tadasana. Finally, bring the hands down.

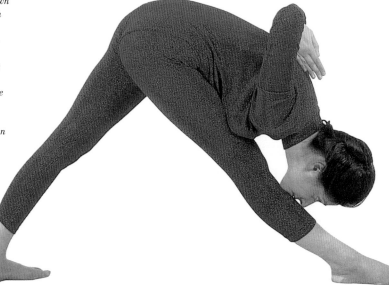

VARIANT (SIMPLE)

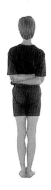

In step 1 (Tadasana), instead of joining the palms behind the back in Namaste, catch the elbows.

VARIANT (WITH ARMS STRETCHED)

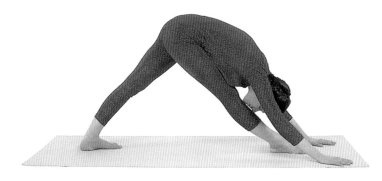

Instead of taking the arms back, stretch them up over the head and then take the trunk and arms down over the leg. Rest the hands on the floor, on either side of the front foot. In this position it is easier to balance and to keep the extension of the trunk.

NAMASTE
HANDS IN PRAYER POSITION

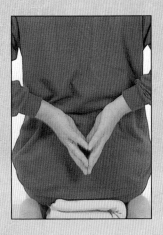

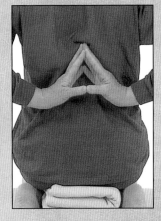

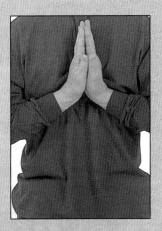

1 *Join the palms behind the back, with the fingers pointing down.*

2 *Turn the hands toward the spine.*

3 *Turn the hands up and raise them between the shoulder blades. Take the shoulders and elbows back and press the palms together.*

8 · PRASARITA PADOTTANASANA
FORWARD STRETCH WITH LEGS WIDE APART

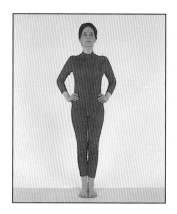

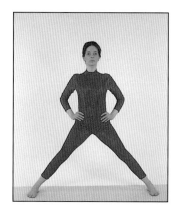

1 Stand in Tadasana (no. 1), with the hands on the hips.

2 With a deep inhalation, jump the feet 4½–5 ft (135–150 cm) apart. Line them up. Turn them to face forward or slightly in so that you do not slip. Straighten the legs and pull up the thigh muscles.

3 *Below: Bend down and place the hands on the floor, shoulder width apart, with the arms slanting back a little. Straighten the arms. Keep the legs firm. Make the back concave and extend the front of the body forward. Look up.*

Bend the elbows back, lower the trunk and place the crown of the head on the floor. If possible take the hands further back, in line with the feet. Lift the hips and the shoulders. Relax and breathe evenly.

Stay for 20–30 seconds. Inhale, raise the head and make the spine concave. Then place the hands on the hips and come up. Bring the feet in a little and jump them together.

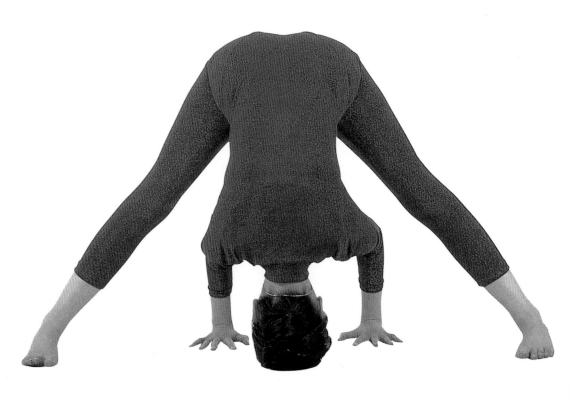

9 · UTTANASANA

FORWARD EXTENSION

Stand in Tadasana (no. 1) with the feet about 1 ft (30 cm) apart. Catch the elbows and take the arms over the head. Draw the waist slightly back. Stretch the legs up strongly.

Exhale and bend down. Bring the hips and chest as close to the legs as possible and if you can, go on extending until the head reaches beyond the knees. Pull on the elbows to bring the trunk further down. Bring the hips further forward to make the legs vertical. Keep the knees straight and the leg muscles pulled up. Relax the head and breathe evenly.

Stay for 20–30 seconds. Inhale, come up and bring the legs together.

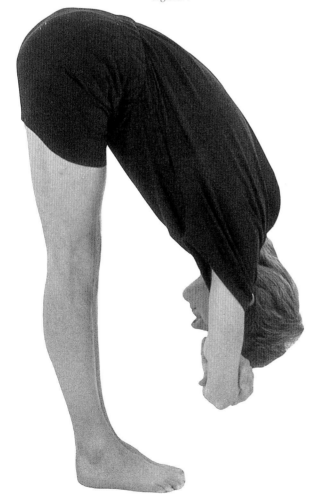

VARIANT (ON LEDGE)

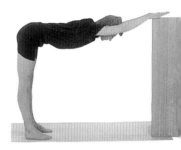

Stand facing a ledge 4–5 ft (120–150 cm) away. Take the feet about 1 ft (30 cm) apart. Bend forward and place the hands on the ledge. Adjust your distance by stepping closer or further away as necessary to enable the legs to be vertical and the trunk and arms to be extended.

Straighten the legs, tighten the kneecaps and pull up the thigh muscles. Extend the arms and the trunk forward. Take the hips further down and make the upper back concave.

Stay for 20–30 seconds.

10 · PADANGUSTHASANA
FINGER-TO-FOOT POSE

11 · GARUDASANA
EAGLE POSE

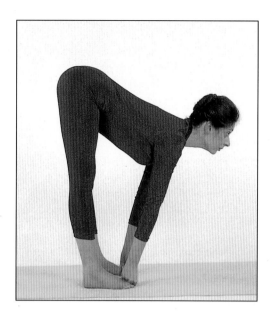

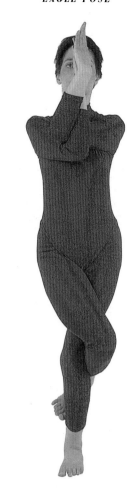

1 Stand with the feet about 1 ft (30 cm) apart. Bend down and make a ring round the big toes with the thumb, index and middle fingers. Straighten the knees and stretch the legs vertically up. Straighten the arms, extend the trunk forward and make the back concave. Look up.

2 Right: Exhale, bend the elbows outward, pull the trunk down and bring the head towards the shins.
  Stay for 20–30 seconds. Inhale and come up, then join the feet and stand erect.

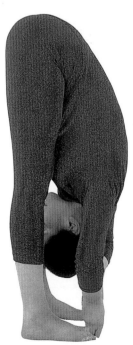

Stand in Tadasana (no. 1). Bend the left leg a little. Bend the right leg and cross the thigh over the left. Swing the right foot back and hook it round the left calf.
  Bend the elbows and raise them to shoulder level, with the thumbs pointing to the face. Cross the left elbow over the right, then hook the right wrist and palm over the left.
  Stay for 20–30 seconds, then repeat on the other side.

12 · UTKATASANA
FIERCE POSE

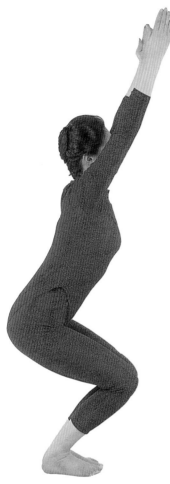

Stand in Tadasana (no. 1). Inhale and stretch the arms over the head, with the palms facing each other. Straighten the elbows and stretch the palms and fingers. Use the hands to pull the trunk up strongly. Bend the knees and take the hips back as if preparing to sit. Bend more in the ankle joints and press the heels down. If you can keep the elbows straight, join the palms.

Stay for 20–30 seconds, then come up.

13 · UTTHITA HASTA PADANGUSTHASANA
LEG RAISING

FORWARD

Stand in Tadasana (no. 1), facing a ledge 2–3 ft (60–90 cm) away. Bend the right leg and place the back of the heel (not the Achilles tendon) on the ledge, directly in front of you. Keep the knee and big toe facing the ceiling. Stretch the left leg and keep the foot facing forward. Straighten both the knees. Extend the right leg and heel away from you. Stretch the left leg and the trunk vertically up. Rest the hands at the sides of the trunk, on the hips or stretch them up.

Stay for 20–30 seconds, then come down and repeat on the other side.

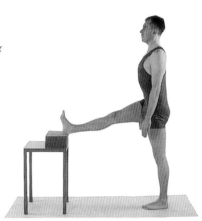

SIDEWAYS

Stand in Tadasana (no. 1), 2–3 ft (60–90 cm) away from a ledge and sideways to it. Bend the right leg outward and place the heel on the ledge, in line with the outer hip. Keep the left leg perpendicular and the foot facing forward. Tighten the kneecaps and the thigh muscles. Stretch the right leg out to the side and stretch the trunk and the left leg upward. Place the hands on the hips or stretch them above the head.

Stay for 20–30 seconds, then take the foot down and repeat on the other side.

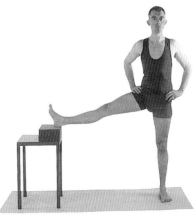

SITTING POSES

14 · SUKHASANA

EASY POSE

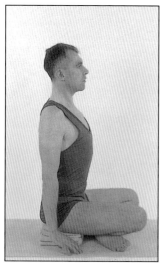

1 *Sit on one or two folded blankets in simple cross-legs. Cross the shins, not only the ankles. Place the hands beside the hips, press the fingertips into the ground and extend the trunk up. Open the chest and take the shoulders back.*

2 *Maintain the trunk erect and bring the hands on to the knees.*
 Stay for 30–60 seconds, then change the cross-legs and repeat.

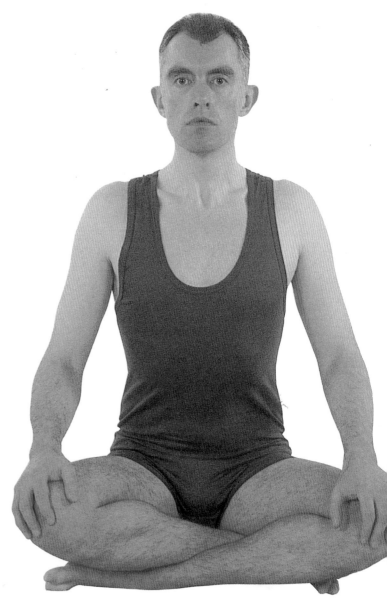

15 · VIRASANA
——— HERO POSE ———

*The knees should be comfortable in this posture. If you
have weak or injured knees, fold a piece of cloth and
place it behind the knee joint to create space; or sit
on a bolster and learn to flex the knees.
For other problems, seek advice.*

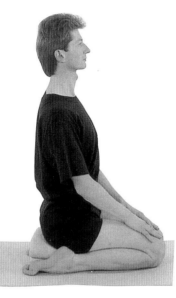

Kneel with the knees together
and the feet apart beside the
hips. Sit between the legs, on a
height of folded blankets if
necessary.

Stretch the trunk up. Take the
shoulders back and broaden
them. Roll the inner thighs
outward to take the outer thighs
down and bring the shins closer
to the thighs. Rest the hands on
the legs.

Stay for 1–2 minutes, then
come out of the posture and
straighten the legs.

16 · VIRASANA FORWARD BEND
——— HERO POSE WITH FORWARD BEND ———

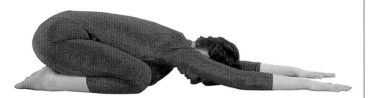

Sit between the legs or on the
heels. If the buttocks do not rest
easily on the heels, place a
folded blanket or bolster on the
heels. Spread the knees slightly
apart and bend down. Stretch the
chest and the arms forward and
keep the sides of the body
touching the inner thighs; do not
spread the legs too wide apart.

17 · PARVATASANA
——— MOUNTAIN POSE ———

*This posture can be done in several
sitting positions, such as
Sukhasana (no. 14) and Virasana
(no. 15).*

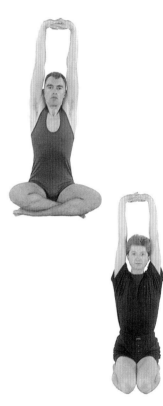

Interlock the fingers. Turn the
palms away from you, stretch the
arms forward and then up over the
head. Do not arch the back at the
waist. Tighten the elbows and
stretch as much as you can.

Stay for 20–30 seconds, then
bring the arms down. Change the
interlock of the fingers (by placing
the right ones in front of the left or
vice versa) and repeat.

18 · DANDASANA
STAFF POSE

Sit on one or two blankets with the legs stretched straight in front of you. Tighten the knees and stretch the feet. Extend the heels and soles, and point the toes up.

Place the palms or fingertips beside the hips and press them down. Stretch the trunk up, paying special attention to lifting the lower back. Extend the spine up from the base. Open the chest to take the shoulders back. Keep the head straight. Relax the eyes and look straight ahead.

Stay for 20–30 seconds, then release.

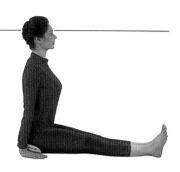

19 · SIDDHASANA
PERFECT POSE

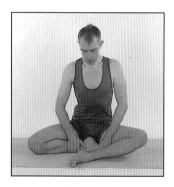

1 Sit in Dandasana (no. 18). Bend the right knee as far to the right as possible, hold the foot from underneath and bring it toward the pubis. Revolve the ankle so that the sole of the foot faces up.

2 Bend the left leg similarly to the left and place the heel on top of the right, sole face up. Tuck in the toes of the left foot between the right thigh and calf and the toes of the right foot between the left thigh and calf. Centre the feet in front of the pubis and open the thighs outward. Stretch the trunk up, especially the lower back. Place the hands on the knees and press them outward, without separating the feet. Maintain a firm posture, with the back straight.

Stay for 30–60 seconds, then change the legs.

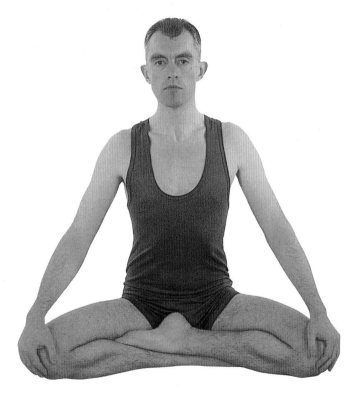

20 · GOMUKHASANA (ARMS ONLY)

HEAD-OF-COW POSE

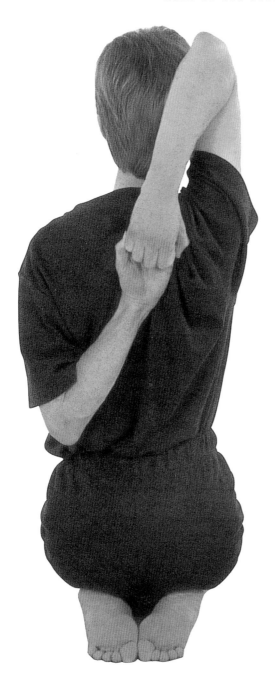

Left: Sit on the heels, or in Virasana (no. 15) or Sukhasana (no. 14). Bend the right arm behind the back, and stretch the hand and forearm up along the spine, with the palm facing out. Bring the elbow in with the other hand.

Stretch the left arm up, turn it so that the palm faces back, then bend the elbow and catch the right hand. Clasp the hands as far as possible. Take the right shoulder back and point the left elbow toward the ceiling. Keep the chest level.

Stay for 30–60 seconds, then repeat on the other side.

VARIANT (STANDING)

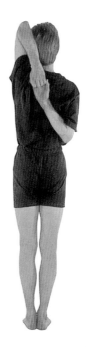

These arm movements can also be done while standing.

21 · JANUSIRSASANA
HEAD-TO-KNEE POSE

● *In case of lower back pain, do not practise the full pose.*

CONCAVE

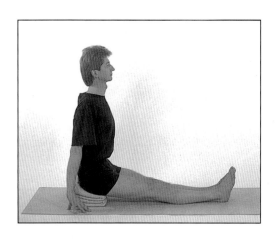

1 *Sit in Dandasana (no. 18) on one or two folded blankets. If your lower back is stiff, you will need more height.*

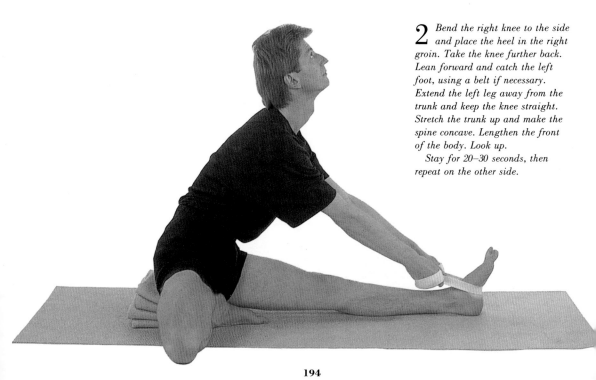

2 *Bend the right knee to the side and place the heel in the right groin. Take the knee further back. Lean forward and catch the left foot, using a belt if necessary. Extend the left leg away from the trunk and keep the knee straight. Stretch the trunk up and make the spine concave. Lengthen the front of the body. Look up.*
   Stay for 20–30 seconds, then repeat on the other side.

FULL POSE

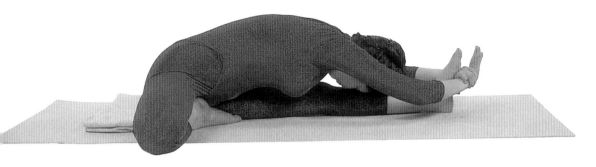

Follow steps 1 and 2. With an
exhalation bend forward over the
left leg. Catch further and take the
head down to the shin.
    Stay for 20–30 seconds, then
repeat on the other side.

VARIANT (HEAD ON
BOLSTER)

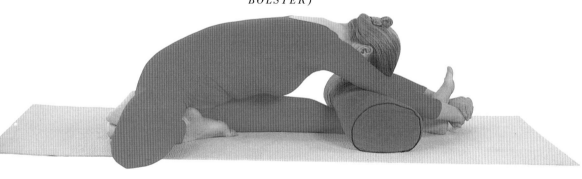

Follow steps 1 and 2. Rest the head
on a folded blanket or bolster.
    Stay for 1–2 minutes, then repeat
on the other side.

● If you are stiff, rest the head on
a stool. If there is strain in the
knee, support it and reduce the
length of time in the posture.

22 · TRIANG MUKHAIKAPADA PASCIMOTTANASANA
FORWARD BEND WITH ONE LEG BENT BACK

CONCAVE

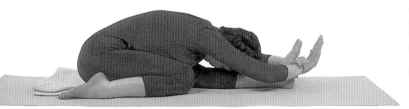

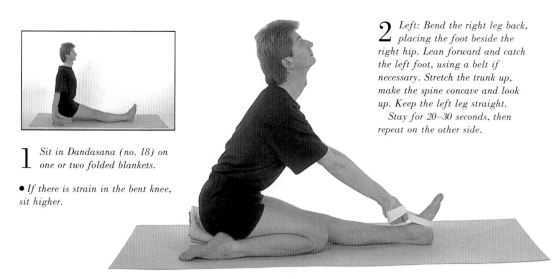

1 Sit in Dandasana (no. 18) on one or two folded blankets.

• If there is strain in the bent knee, sit higher.

2 Left: Bend the right leg back, placing the foot beside the right hip. Lean forward and catch the left foot, using a belt if necessary. Stretch the trunk up, make the spine concave and look up. Keep the left leg straight.
   Stay for 20–30 seconds, then repeat on the other side.

FULL POSE

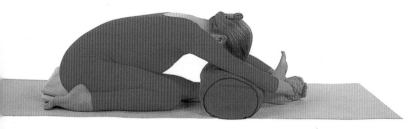

Follow steps 1 and 2 above. With an exhalation, bend forward over the left leg. Elongate the trunk and catch further. Take the head down.
   Stay for 20–30 seconds, then repeat on the other side.

VARIANT (HEAD ON BOLSTER)

Follow steps 1 and 2 above. Rest the head on a blanket or bolster.
   Stay for 1–2 minutes, then repeat on the other side.

• If you are stiff, rest the head on a stool.

23 · MARICYASANA I (TWIST ONLY)

SIMPLE TWIST CATCHING THE ARMS BEHIND

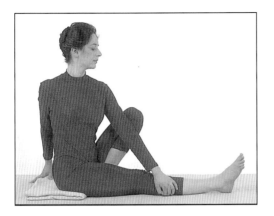

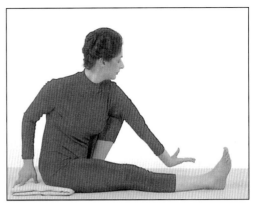

1 *Sit in Dandasana (no. 18) on one or two folded blankets. Bend the left knee up and bring the foot in front of the pubis. Place the inner edge of the foot against the right inner thigh. Keep the right leg extended. Turn to the right, and bring the left upper arm in front of the left knee. Place the right hand beside the right hip.*

2 *Press the fingertips of the right hand into the floor, and the left arm against the left knee, to turn the trunk more. Rotate the left arm inward so that the palm faces back.*

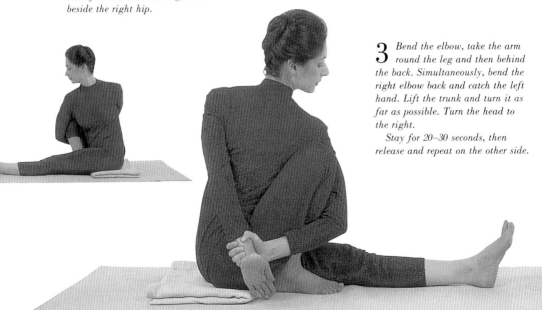

3 *Bend the elbow, take the arm round the leg and then behind the back. Simultaneously, bend the right elbow back and catch the left hand. Lift the trunk and turn it as far as possible. Turn the head to the right.*
   Stay for 20–30 seconds, then release and repeat on the other side.

24 · PASCIMOTTANASANA
FULL FORWARD BEND

CONCAVE

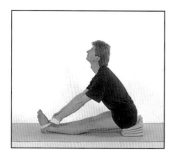

Sit in Dandasana (no. 18) on one or two folded blankets. Lean forward and catch the feet, using a belt if necessary. Stretch the trunk up. Make the back concave, lift the chest and look up. Keep the knees straight.

Stay for 20–30 seconds, then release.

FULL POSE

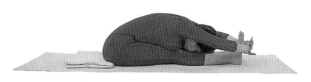

Follow the method as above, then bend forward over the legs, catching further with the hands. Stretch the front of the body and the spine to go further. Maintain an even extension of both legs and both sides of the body. Take the head down.

Stay for 20–30 seconds, then come up.

VARIANT (HEAD ON BOLSTER)

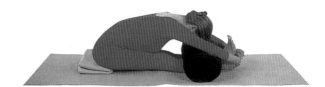

Do the posture as above, resting the head on a bolster or blankets. Quieten the mind. Stay for 2–3 minutes, then come up.

25 · MALASANA (PREPARATORY)
GARLAND POSE

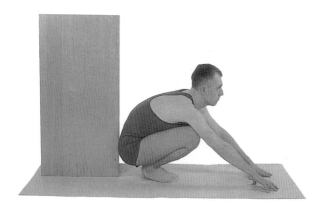

Squat, leaning the lower back against a wall. Keep the heels down if possible. Spread the knees apart but keep the feet together. Take the trunk down between the thighs and knees. Stretch the arms and chest forward, with the hands on the floor.

Stay for 30–60 seconds, then stand up.

SUPINE AND PRONE POSES

26 · CROSS BOLSTERS

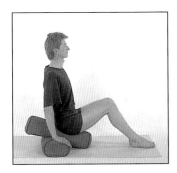

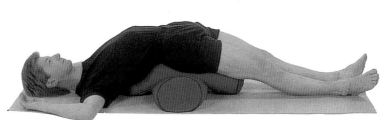

1 *Arrange two bolsters as a cross on the floor, with the lengthwise one on top. Sit on the bolsters.*

2 *Lie back and stretch the legs forward. Place the lower back on the highest part of the bolster arrangement and the shoulders on the floor. You can tie the thighs together with a belt for a passive extension and to make the posture more restful. Take the arms over the* head *and relax. If the lower back feels pinched, pass the hands underneath it from waist to buttocks to lengthen and ease it.*

Stay for 3–5 minutes. To get up, slide back a little toward the head, then bend the knees and turn to the side.

27 · MATSYASANA (SIMPLE)
——— FISH POSE ———

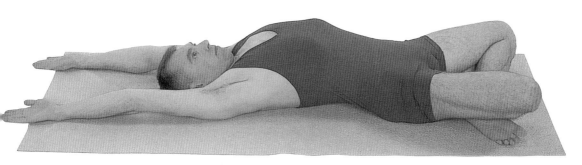

Sit in Sukhasana (no. 14). Lean back and lie down. While lying down, extend the lower back. Take the arms over the head and straighten the elbows. Stretch the whole trunk, especially the abdominal area.

Stay for 1–2 minutes, then come up, change the cross-legs and repeat.

28 · SUPTA BADDHAKONASANA
LYING DOWN IN BADDHAKONASANA

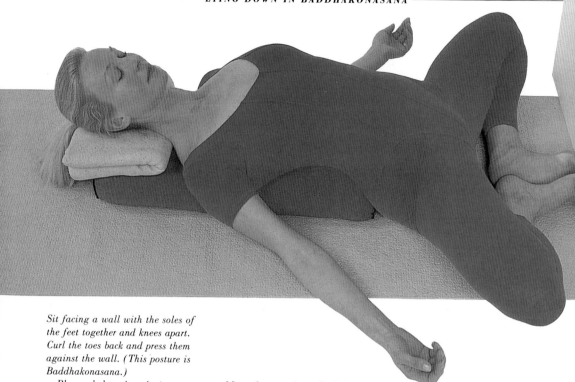

Sit facing a wall with the soles of
the feet together and knees apart.
Curl the toes back and press them
against the wall. (This posture is
Baddhakonasana.)

Place a bolster lengthwise
behind the lower back, hold it
toward you and lie back over it,
with the shoulders on the ground.

Move closer to the wall. Take the
arms over the head. Breathe evenly.
Stay for 2–5 minutes. Turn to the
side to get up.

• If your legs are uncomfortable,
place a blanket under the thighs.

29 · SUPTA VIRASANA
RECLINING HERO POSE

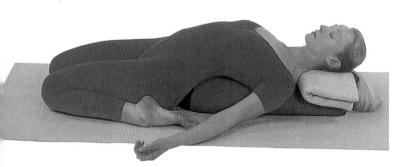

Sit in Virasana (no. 15). Place a
bolster (or folded blankets) behind
you. Hold it against the lower back
and lie down. Place an extra
blanket under the head if necessary.
Relax. Stay for 3–5 minutes, then
get up.

• If you need to sit on something in
Virasana you will also need a high
support under the back.

30 · URDHVA PRASARITA PADASANA

LEGS STRETCHED TO 90°

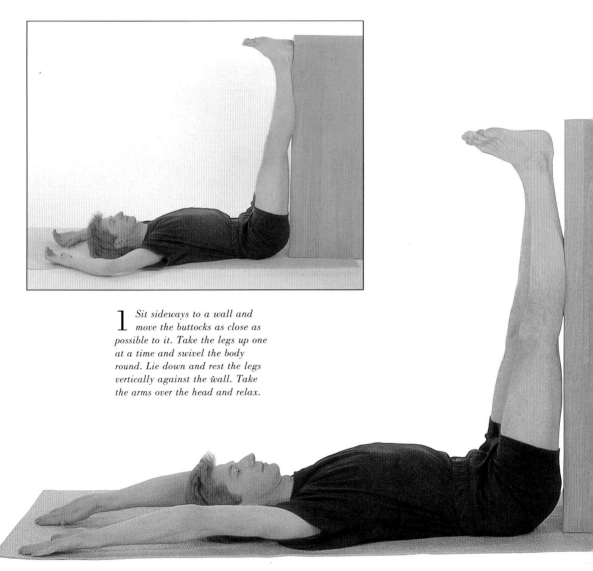

1 Sit sideways to a wall and move the buttocks as close as possible to it. Take the legs up one at a time and swivel the body round. Lie down and rest the legs vertically against the wall. Take the arms over the head and relax.

2 Keeping the hips down, straighten the legs and stretch them up. Stretch the arms over the head.

Stay for 20–30 seconds (or longer). To come down, bend the knees and turn to the side.

31 · ADHO MUKHA SVANASANA
— DOG POSE —

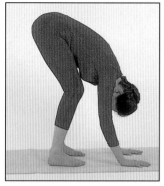

2 *Below: Step about 3–4 ft (90–120 cm) back and straighten the legs, so that the body makes an inverted "V" shape. Lift up the hips, press the thighs back and extend the heels downward.*

Straighten the elbows, *lift the shoulders and stretch the trunk up. Keep the arms and legs firm. Relax the head.*

Stay for 20–30 seconds, then bend the knees and come down.

1 *Stand in Tadasana (no. 1). Take the feet hip-width apart. Bend down and place the palms on the floor in front of the feet and shoulder-width apart. Spread the fingers.*

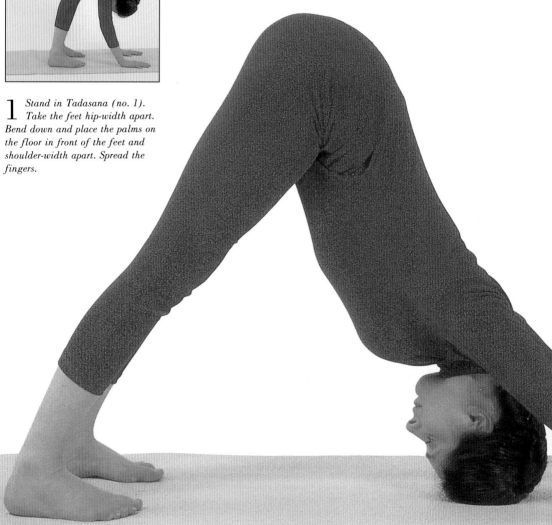

VARIANT (HEAD SUPPORTED)

1 *Right: Place a folded blanket or bolster lengthwise a short distance from the wall. Kneel in front of it. Place the hands, palms down, near the wall. Touch the wall with the thumbs and index fingers, spreading them as far apart as possible.*

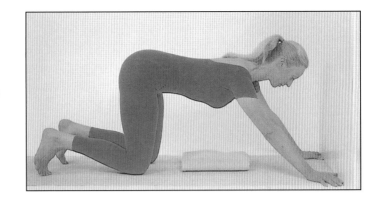

2 *Below: Raise the hips and straighten the legs. Rest the head on the blanket. Stretch the arms and trunk up strongly. Do not let the weight of the body sink on to the head. Relax the head.*
   Stay for 30–60 seconds, then come down.

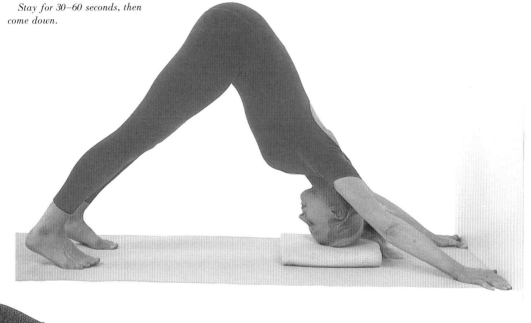

TWISTING POSES

32 · MARICYASANA (STANDING)

—— STANDING TWIST ——

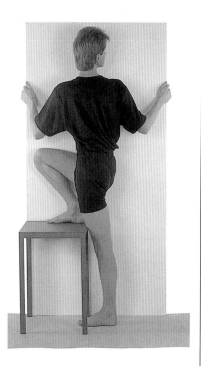

Place a high stool or small table near a wall or ledge. Stand in Tadasana (no. 1) with the right side of the body by the wall. Raise the right foot on to the stool and press the foot down. Keep the right thigh touching the wall. Stretch the trunk up and turn toward the wall, holding on with the hands wherever possible to give you leverage. Keep the left leg and trunk vertical, and the foot facing forward. Turn as far as you can.

Stay for 20–30 seconds, come down and repeat on the other side.

33 · BHARADVAJASANA

—— SIMPLE TWIST ——

PREPARATORY

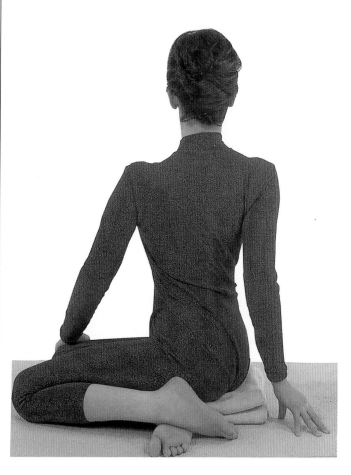

Sit in Dandasana (no. 18) on one or two folded blankets. Bend the legs to the left. Place the left foot on top of the right instep, with the sole of the left foot facing up. Extend the spine and the trunk up. Turn to the right. Place the left hand on the outer side of the right knee and the right hand beside the right hip. Use the arms to help turn the trunk. Turn the hips, waist and chest as far as you can.

Stay for 20–30 seconds. Turn to the front, and repeat on the other side.

FULL POSE

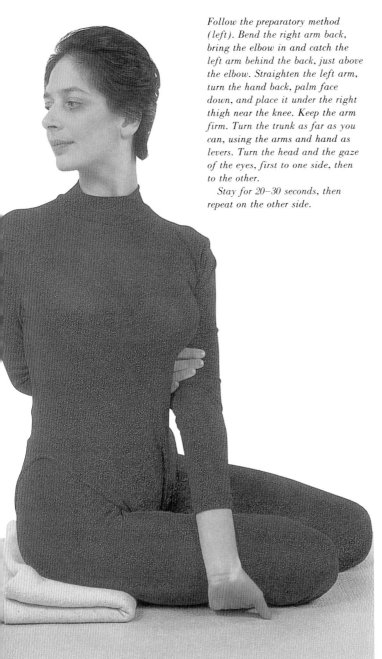

Follow the preparatory method (left). Bend the right arm back, bring the elbow in and catch the left arm behind the back, just above the elbow. Straighten the left arm, turn the hand back, palm face down, and place it under the right thigh near the knee. Keep the arm firm. Turn the trunk as far as you can, using the arms and hand as levers. Turn the head and the gaze of the eyes, first to one side, then to the other.

Stay for 20–30 seconds, then repeat on the other side.

VARIANT (ON A CHAIR)

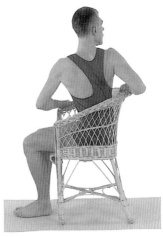

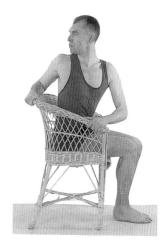

Sit on a chair, with the knees and feet together. Lift the hips, waist and ribcage. Turn to the right, holding the back of the chair. Keep the trunk vertical and lifted and turn to the maximum. Turn the head and neck to the right.

Stay for 20–30 seconds, then repeat on the other side.

INVERTED POSES

34 · SARVANGASANA
NECK BALANCE

1 *Prepare a set of four or five folded blankets, with the folded edges neatly together. The height should be 2–3 inches (5–7.5 cm), the width sufficient for the shoulders, and the depth enough to accommodate the length of the upper arms. If the arms and elbows slip apart, tie a belt round the upper arms, just above the elbows, approximately shoulder width apart.*

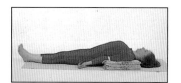

Lie down with the shoulders on the blankets, 2–3 inches (5–7.5 cm) away from the edge, and the head on the floor. Check that you are in a straight line.

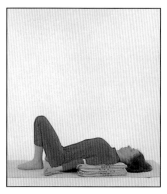

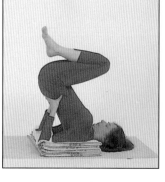

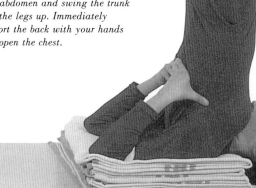

2 *Flex the knees and bring the feet toward the buttocks. Then lift the lower back slightly and lengthen it away from you.*

3 *Bend the knees over the abdomen and swing the trunk and the legs up. Immediately support the back with your hands and open the chest.*

4 *Straighten the legs up. Move the hands further up the back towards the shoulder blades to give you maximum lift and support. Bring the chest toward the chin. Stretch the whole body up. Keep the posture stable.*

Stay for 2–5 minutes. To come down, bend the legs and slide down.

35 · HALASANA
PLOUGH POSE

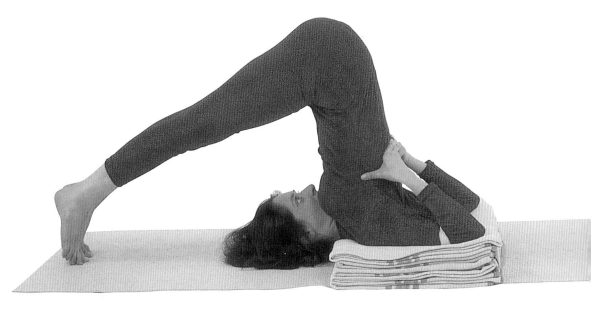

NOTE

- Inverted poses should not be practised during menstruation.
- If you experience pressure in the head, eyes, ears or throat in any inverted pose, come down and rest. Then seek advice.

From Sarvangasana (no. 34) take the legs down over the head and rest the feet on the floor. Keep the hands on the back, lift the trunk and extend front of the body up. Straighten the knees and stretch the legs away from the hips. Relax the face, the eyes and the ears.

Stay for 2–5 minutes, then slide down.

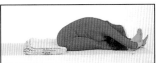

- If you wish, after sliding down from Halasana, sit on the edge of the blanket and rest forward in Pascimottanasana (no. 24).

36 · ARDHA HALASANA
HALF PLOUGH POSE

Place a chair or stool over the head before you go up into Sarvangasana (no. 34). From Sarvangasana take the legs down on to the chair to support the thighs.

Take the arms over the head and relax. Do not let the shoulders slip off the blankets.

Stay for 3–5 minutes. Come down with bent knees and ease yourself off the stool, at the same time pushing it away with the hands. Slide down.

- If you have a long trunk you may increase the height by placing a bolster or blankets on the stool.
- If your back is very stiff, keep the stool further away and support the shins.
- If the neck hurts, increase the height of the blankets.

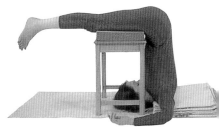

37 · SARVANGASANA (ON CHAIR)

NECK BALANCE

Use a sturdy armchair that will not topple. Take each stage slowly and carefully, so that you feel secure.

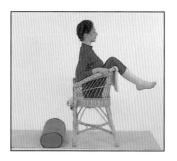

1 *Place a bolster crosswise on the floor in front of the armchair. Sit facing the back of the chair, with the legs bent over the back of it and holding on to the sides.*

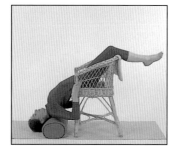

3 *Lean back further so that the waist curves over the edge of the seat and the head goes down.*

4 *Below: Rest the shoulders on the bolster. Straighten the legs and stretch them against the back of the chair. Depending on the construction of the chair, hold the chair or take the arms over the head. Keep the back ribs tucked in and the chest open.*

Stay for 5–8 minutes, then come down as shown in steps 5–7.

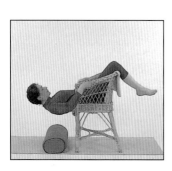

2 *Move the hips closer to the back of the chair, hold the arms and lean back.*

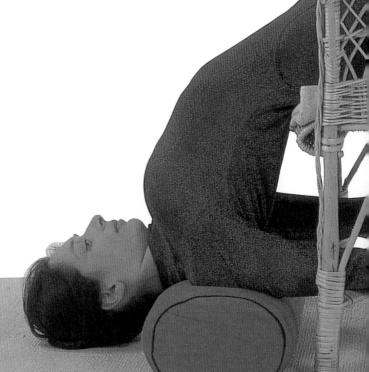

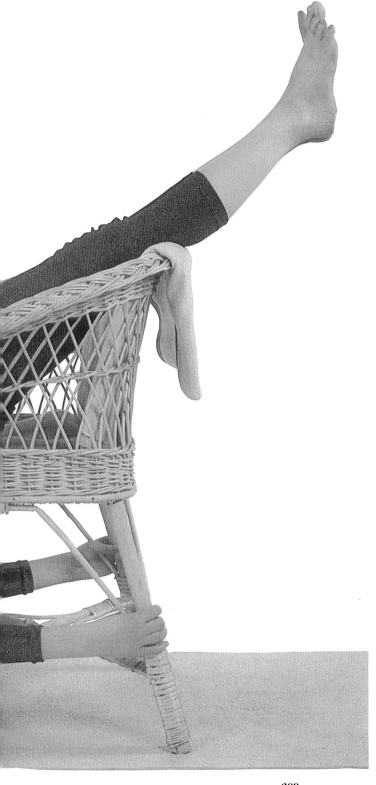

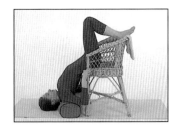

5 *Bend the legs and place the feet on the back of the armchair. Hold the arms of the chair.*

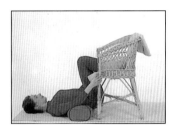

6 *Slide backward off the armchair till the lower back rests on the bolster. Stay for a moment.*

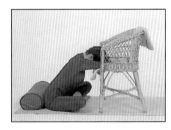

7 *Turn to the side, sit cross-legged in front of the chair and rest your head on it.*

You may need to experiment with bolsters and blankets to obtain the height you need.

38 · SARVANGASANA (AGAINST WALL)

NECK BALANCE AGAINST WALL

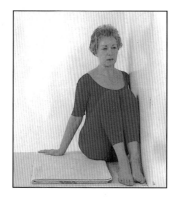

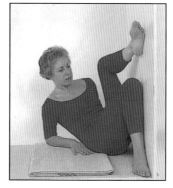

5 *Below: Support the back with the hands and bring the elbows in. Straighten the legs, keeping the feet on the wall. Lift the chest, abdomen and hips. Breathe evenly. Stay for 3–5 minutes, then bend the legs and come down.*

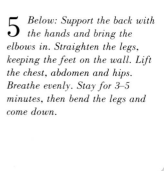

1 *Place one or two folded blankets near a wall, with the folded edges away from it. Sit on them sideways, as close to the wall as possible.*

2 *Lean back on to the elbows, swivel the trunk round and take one leg up the wall.*

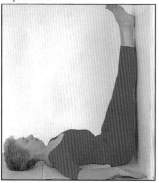

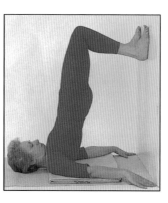

3 *Take the other leg up the wall and lie back. Place the buttocks against the wall, the shoulders on the blankets, and the head on the floor.*

4 *Bend the legs, press the feet against the wall and raise the hips and chest.*

39 · SETU BANDHA SARVANGASANA (SUPPORTED)

— NECK BALANCE BACK ARCH —

This posture may be done during menstruation. To make the pose more restful, tie a belt round the middle thighs.

| ON BOLSTER | ON BENCH |

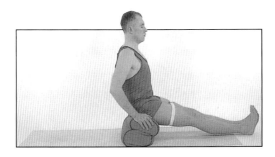

1   *Place two bolsters on top of each other horizontally on the floor and sit on them.*

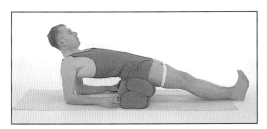

2   *Slide slightly back so that the lower back is nearly off the bolster.*

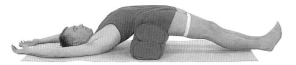

3   *Support yourself on your arms. Lie back with the shoulders and head on the floor. Take the arms over the head and relax. Stay for 5–8 minutes.*

● *If the lower back feels pinched, stretch it away from the waist or raise the feet and support them.*
● *To come down, bend the knees, push the bolsters away and slide back. Remove the belt (if used). Turn to the side, then sit cross-legged in front of the bolsters and bend forward, resting the head on them.*

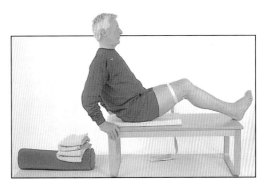

1   *Place one or two blankets on a sturdy bench. Place a bolster lengthwise on the floor in front of it. Sit backwards near the edge of the bench and take the feet up on to it.*

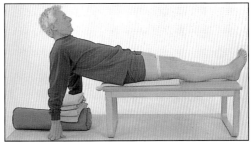

2   *Place the hands on the floor. Lean back, curving the waist over the edge of the bench. Straighten the legs.*

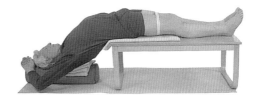

3   *Rest the shoulders and head on the bolster. Take the arms over the head. Stay for 5–8 minutes.*

40 · VIPARITA KARANI
RESTFUL INVERSION

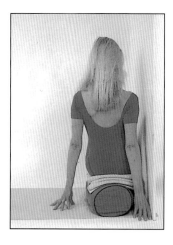

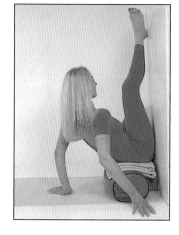

1 *Place a block or thick book against the wall, with a bolster in front of it. Place one or more folded blankets on top, depending on your height. Sit sideways on the bolster, with the right hip touching the wall.*

2 *With the help of the hands, swivel the body round and take the right leg up the wall. Keep the right buttock against the wall.*

3 *Continue to swivel the body round and take the left leg up. At the same time lean back till the shoulders and head reach the floor. Support the lower back on the bolster arrangement and rest the buttocks and legs against the wall. Take the arms over the head and relax.*

Stay for 5-8 minutes. Bend the knees, slide back, turn to the side and get up.

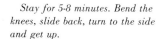

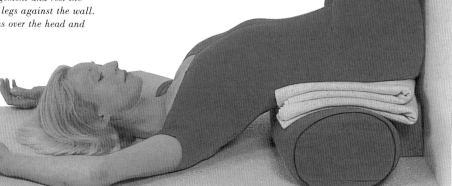

RELAXATION

41 · SAVASANA

CORPSE POSE

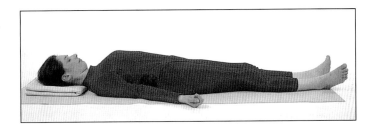

Lie on the floor in a straight line, with the feet together. Line yourself up carefully, as any lack of alignment prevents you from relaxing completely. Stretch the arms and legs and then relax them. Keep the arms slightly away from the trunk, with the palms facing up. Allow the legs and feet to roll away from each other.

Place a blanket under the head and neck at a comfortable height, so that the forehead and chin do not tilt backward. Close the eyes and let go mentally. Observe whether you are lying evenly on the floor. Feel the weight of the body sinking into the floor and the mind becoming quiet. Breathe evenly.

Stay for 5–10 minutes. To get up, slowly open the eyes, bend the knees and turn to the side.

VARIANT (ON A BOLSTER)

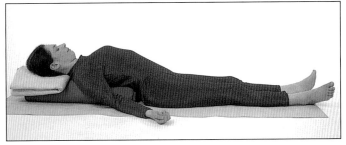

Place a bolster or two narrowly folded blankets lengthwise on the floor. Sit in front of the bolster and hold it against your back. Lean back and lie down on it. Centre the spine on it. Place a folded blanket under the head. Press the shoulders down and away from the neck. Move the back of the head away from the shoulders. Stretch the arms and legs away from the trunk and then relax them. Relax the hands and fingers, palms face up. Extend the soles of the feet and the toes, then let the feet drop to the sides.

Close the eyes and relax. Breathe quietly and enjoy the feeling of the chest opening with the support of the bolster.

Stay for 5–10 minutes. Before getting up slowly open the eyes, bend the knees and turn to the side.

When Savasana is done on a bolster, the mind and body relax well as the chest is open, and breathing comes easily. The posture strengthens the lungs and is thus a good preparation for pranayama.

TOWARD MENTAL PEACE

Pranayama is control of the breath, from the subtlest to the most complex level. According to Patanjali it is not to be attempted until practice of the postures is mastered and, according to orthodox tradition, it is not to be attempted except under expert supervision.

The purpose of the postures and breathing exercises is the development of a sound and healthy body and mind. Yoga philosophy insists that this must be achieved before a person can embark on a programme of philosophical and spiritual development.

Without the one, the other is not possible. But when the foundation is firm, progress is assured.

RELAXING THE BODY

Lie on a bolster in Savasana (no. 41, variant). Spend a few minutes relaxing the body. Release tension from the feet and legs, the arms and hands, the abdomen and the face. Still your thoughts.

Keep the eyes quiet. Let the eyeballs sink down into the eye-sockets. Relax the temples and the forehead. Relax the skin at the bridge of the nose. Relax the cheeks by releasing them away from the eyes. Relax the jaws, moving the lower jaw a little away from the upper, without tensing it. Quieten the ears. Feel the connection between the ear passages and the jaws and relax them. Keep the tongue still. Let it rest on the lower palate and as it relaxes, allow the root of the tongue to recede into the throat. Do not clench the teeth; keep them very slightly parted.

Relax the neck and throat. If you cannot relax them, press the shoulders down and move the shoulder-blades into the back ribs. At the same time bring the chin slightly down towards the throat. Quieten the vibrations of the vocal cords.

In the early stages of your practice, end your relaxation here. Lie flat on your back, then bend the legs and turn to the side before getting up.

OBSERVING THE BREATH

Spend about five minutes relaxing on a bolster as described above.

When the body feels relaxed, begin to observe your breathing. Take the gaze of the eyes downward and then inward into the chest. Follow the course of the breath. Do not alter it, but watch the rhythm of your normal breathing. Observe whether you are breathing evenly and equally in both nostrils. Observe the speed of the breath, and whether your inhalations and exhalations are the same length. Keep your breathing soft and quiet.

Continue in the same way for a few minutes. As you watch the breath, do not lose the awareness of your relaxation. Maintain the quiet state of the body from moment to moment.

Relaxation needs to be learned. You will find that while you are concentrating on the breath,

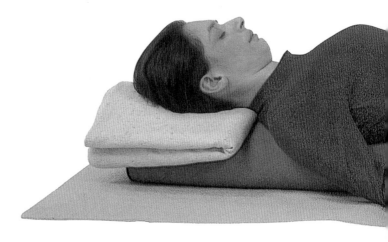

tension creeps into different parts of the body. Some areas of tension are common to everyone. During inhalation, everyone has the habit of moving the head backward and lifting the chin; move them back to their original position every time. Similarly, tension returns unconsciously to the hands and feet, and the abdomen. Release this tension as soon as you observe it, during exhalation.

Other areas of tension in the body are individual, depending on each person's physique and habitual posture. Injuries, stiffness and the asymmetrical development of muscles and joints all prevent the free flow of energy and relaxation in the body. So too do mental and emotional strain. This is why the practice of postures is necessary: they counteract the wear and tear of daily life.

Relaxation and pranayama go one step further by training the mind to look inward. They induce a state of calmness that can be experienced again and again. This develops a reserve of inner strength.

The next stage of your relaxation can end here for the first few weeks of practice. When you have gained more experience you may continue by deeping your relaxation (see overleaf).

PREPARATORY PRANAYAMA TEN-WEEK COURSE

Sundays in the ten-week course are devoted to relaxing poses. Pranayama preparation can be added to these in the following way:

WEEKS 1 & 2	*Relaxing the Body*
WEEKS 3 & 4	*Observing the Breath*
WEEK 5	Repeat weeks 1–4
WEEKS 6 & 7	*Deepening your Relaxation* Add: *Normal Inhalation, Lengthened Exhalation* and *Lengthened Inhalation, Normal Inhalation*
WEEKS 8 & 9	*Deepening your Relaxation* Add: *Lengthened Inhalation and Exhalation*
WEEK 10	Repeat any of the techniques given in weeks 6–9.

Below: For relaxation practice, lie on a bolster in Savasana (no. 41, variant), opening the chest well. Ensure that you are settled comfortably so there is no physical distraction from your relaxation.

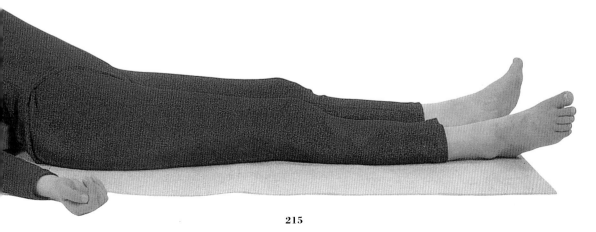

DEEPENING RELAXATION

After spending a few minutes observing your normal breathing, practise the following technique for lengthening the breath.

Normal Inhalation, Lengthened Exhalation

First exhale and relax the abdomen. Inhale normally. Exhale slowly and quietly. Do not strain. Again take a normal inhalation, then exhale slowly and quietly.

Continue in this way for about five minutes. Then lie quietly and breathe normally. Enjoy lying down and relaxing. Allow a few minutes to elapse before continuing.

Lengthened Inhalation, Normal Exhalation

Exhale completely, then take a slow, quiet inhalation. Do not breathe in suddenly or deeply, but lengthen the breath smoothly. Exhale normally. Again inhale slowly and quietly, taking care not to tense the eyes or brain. Do not let the breath disturb the nostrils. Exhale normally.

Continue in this way for about five minutes. Then lie quietly and breathe normally.

Allow a few minutes to elapse before continuing.

This is enough breathing practice for the first few sessions.

Lengthened Inhalations and Exhalations

Exhale completely, to empty the lungs of stale air and to prepare yourself psychologically. Inhale slowly and quietly, lengthening the breath as above. Do not hurry. Then exhale slowly and softly, lengthening the breath as above. Relax completely. Again take a quiet, slow inhalation, without tensing, and then a quiet, slow exhalation.

Continue for about five minutes, then breathe normally.

ENDING YOUR RELAXATION

Bend the legs, turn to the side, remove the bolster from under you, and lie flat on the back in Savasana. Keep the blanket for the head. Settle down on the floor; keep the mind quiet. Let go completely. Relax the brain. Move the awareness down into the chest.

Then carefully open the eyes, bend the knees and turn to the right side. Stay for a little while, then turn to the left. Get up from the side, or from the front.

Below: Savasana (no. 41) without a bolster is used for the final stage of relaxation practice. Check that your body is in alignment and lie still, keeping the mind and body quiet.

CONCLUSION

If Patanjali's teachings are followed and the inner body and the mind and nervous system are strengthened through asana practice, then the beginning stages of pranayama may safely be practised. However, it is preferable to have an experienced teacher to guide you in the early stages. Traditionally, it was considered essential to have a guru.

Until relaxation is learnt thoroughly, and the lungs are trained to alter their breathing pattern without strain, pranayama, the control of the breath, cannot be learnt. This is why, traditionally, it is not taught to beginners. One yoga text says that learning to control the breath is like learning to tame a tiger. The "father" of yoga, Patanjali, says that the practice of asanas must be mastered first.

The explanations of yoga in this book are aimed to be a guide to the first steps of yoga practice. The end of yoga is meditation and spiritual awareness. These refined mental and spiritual states cannot be experienced without due preparation. The path is acknowledged to be long, but the benefits at every step are so great that countless people, of former ages and today, have found the effort worthwhile.

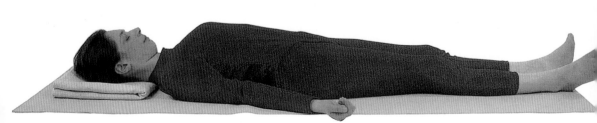

TOOLS FOR PRACTICE

In the Iyengar method props and equipment are used in yoga practice when the body cannot achieve a posture or make a particular effort to achieve a required result of its own accord. This principle is important in yoga therapy, but is also useful when practising generally.

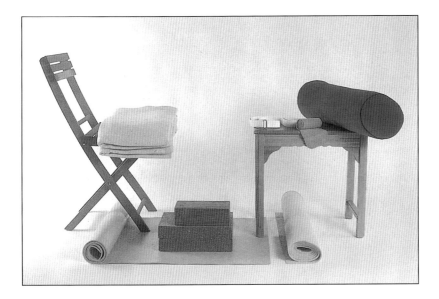

Most of the items required are common equipment found in a home. If the exact "prop" is not available, it can usually be substituted by something else.

Supporting the body in the asanas enables muscular extensions to be done in a passive way. It also helps to improve blood circulation and respiratory capacity.

The items used in this book are:

- **Armchair** For supported Sarvangasana (no. 37).
- **Bandage** In forward bends, to wind round the forehead.
- **Belt** In Sarvangasana (no. 34), to keep the elbows in.
In forward bends, to help catch the foot.
- **Bench** For Setu Bandha Sarvangasana (no. 39) to arch the back and open the chest.
- **Blankets** For Sarvangasana (no. 34) and Halasana (no. 35), to prevent compression of the neck.

For sitting poses, to lift the lower back.
For Savasana (no. 41), to support the head.
- **Block/Brick** In standing poses, to support the lower hand when it is difficult to reach the floor.
- **Bolsters** In supine poses, to support the back and lift the chest.
- **Chair** In twists, to facilitate the turning of the spine to the maximum.
- **Door Post** For Supta Padangusthasana, to support the raised leg.

- **Ledge** In standing poses and twists, to allow an effective grip, enabling the body to turn.
- **Non-slip Mat** To prevent slipping in standing poses, etc.
- **Pole** In Uttanasana (no. 9), to increase the shoulder movement.
- **Stool** In Ardha Halasana (no. 36), to support the thighs for a restful pose.
In standing twists and leg raisings, to support the lifted leg.
- **Wall** In standing poses and twists, to give support and a sense of direction.

TEN-WEEK COURSE

The course consists of 41 postures (asanas) and their variants. Dynamic and relaxing poses are given on alternate days so that the body experiences a balance of effort and recuperation. As strength, stamina and suppleness increase, more postures are added.

The course is intended only as a guide to structuring your practice. Basic instructions for the postures are given in the Asana section. If at all possible, it is advisable to attend a class with a teacher as well as following the course.

The course is devised for daily practice, of approximately 30 minutes to one hour each day. It can be adapted or spread out according to individual need and circumstances.

The number of the postures refer to their sequence in the Asana section, an asterisk indicates that a posture is being introduced for the first time.

WEEK 1

MONDAY

- *1 • Tadasana
- *2 • Vrksasana
- *3 • Trikonasana
- *4 • Parsvakonasana
- *6 • Virabhadrasana II
- *9 • Uttanasana (on ledge)
- *16 • Virasana (forward bend)
- *14 • Sukhasana
- *41 • Savasana

TUESDAY AND THURSDAY

- 9 • Uttanasana (on ledge)
- *31 • Adho Mukha Svanasana (head supported)
- 14 • Sukhasana
- *17 • Parvatasana (in Sukhasana)
- *20 • Gomukhasana (arms only)
- *39 • Setu Bandha Sarvangasana (on bolster)
- *40 • Viparita Karani
- 41 • Savasana

WEDNESDAY AND FRIDAY

- 1 • Tadasana
- 2 • Vrksasana
- 3 • Trikonasana
- 4 • Parsvakonasana
- 6 • Virabhadrasana II
- 9 • Uttanasana (on ledge)
- 16 • Virasana (forward bend)
- 14 • Sukhasana
- *34 • Sarvangasana
- 41 • Savasana

SATURDAY

- 1 • Tadasana
- 2 • Vrksasana
- 3 • Trikonasana
- 4 • Parsvakonasana
- 6 • Virabhadrasana II
- 9 • Uttanasana (on ledge)
- 16 • Virasana (forward bend)
- *15 • Virasana
- 14 • Sukhasana
- 17 • Parvatasana (in Sukhasana)
- 20 • Gomukhasana
- 34 • Sarvangasana
- *36 • Ardha Halasana
- 41 • Savasana

SUNDAY

- *26 • Cross Bolsters
- *27 • Matsyasana (simple)
- 31 • Adho Mukha Svanasana (head supported)
- *9 • Uttanasana
- 39 • Setu Bandha Sarvangasana (on bolster)
- 40 • Viparita Karani
- *41 • Savasana (on bolster)

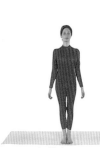

1 · Tadasana

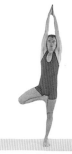

2 · Vrksasana

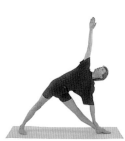

3 · Trikonasana

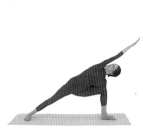

4 · Parsvakonasana

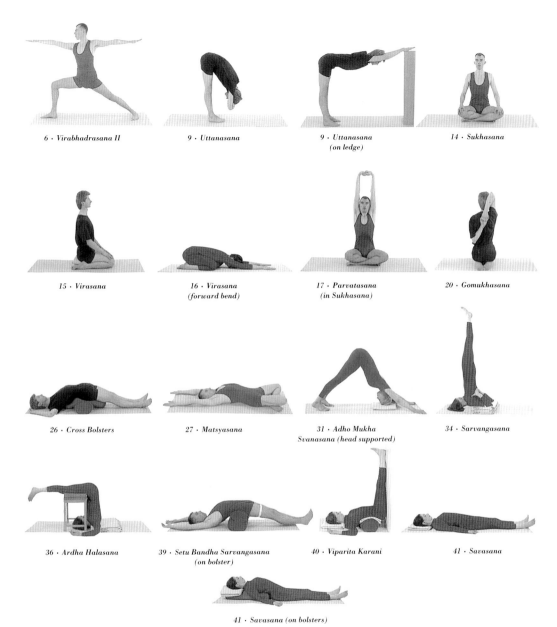

6 · Virabhadrasana II

9 · Uttanasana

9 · Uttanasana
(on ledge)

14 · Sukhasana

15 · Virasana

16 · Virasana
(forward bend)

17 · Parvatasana
(in Sukhasana)

20 · Gomukhasana

26 · Cross Bolsters

27 · Matsyasana

31 · Adho Mukha
Svanasana (head supported)

34 · Sarvangasana

36 · Ardha Halasana

39 · Setu Bandha Sarvangasana
(on bolster)

40 · Viparita Karani

41 · Savasana

41 · Savasana (on bolsters)

POINTS TO PRACTISE

Standing Poses

● Stand evenly on the inner and outer edges of the feet, and on the heels and mounds of the toes.

● Stretch the toes.
● Tighten the knees and pull up the thigh muscles.
● Keep the back leg strong and stable while bending the front leg.
● Make a right angle accurately.

● In turned poses, turn the hips to the maximum.
● Open the palms and extend fingers.
● Turn the head and neck without straining.
● Keep the face relaxed.

219

WEEK 2

MONDAY, WEDNESDAY AND FRIDAY

1 · *Tadasana*
3 · *Trikonasana*
4 · *Parsvakonasana*
6 · *Virabhadrasana II*
*7 · *Parsvottanasana* (simple)*
9 · *Uttanasana*
*31 · *Adho Mukha Svanasana*
16 · *Virasana* (forward bend)*
34 · *Sarvangasana*
*35 · *Halasana*
41 · *Savasana*

TUESDAY AND THURSDAY

*33 · *Bharadvajasana* (on chair)*
14 · *Sukhasana*
17 · *Parvatasana* (in Sukhasana)*
*15 · *Virasana*
*17 · *Parvatasana* (in Virasana)*
20 · *Gomukhasana* (arms only)*
31 · *Adho Mukha Svanasana*
34 · *Sarvangasana*
35 · *Halasana*
41 · *Savasana*

SATURDAY

31 · *Adho Mukha Svanasana*
9 · *Uttanasana* (on ledge)*
1 · *Tadasana*
2 · *Vrksasana*
3 · *Trikonasana*
4 · *Parsvakonasana*
6 · *Virabhadrasana II*
*7 · *Parsvottanasana* (full pose)*
16 · *Virasana* (forward bend)*
34 · *Sarvangasana*
35 · *Halasana*
41 · *Savasana*

SUNDAY

26 · *Cross Bolsters*
27 · *Matsyasana* (simple)*
31 · *Adho Mukha Svanasana* (head supported)*
9 · *Uttanasana*
39 · *Setu Bandha Sarvangasana* (on bolster)*
40 · *Viparita Karani*
41 · *Savasana* (on bolster)*

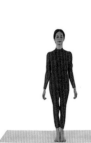

1 · Tadasana

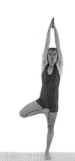

2 · Vrksasana

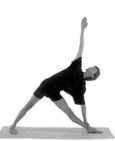

3 · Trikonasana

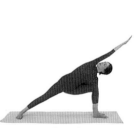

4 · Parsvakonasana

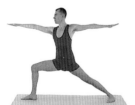

6 · Virabhadrasana II

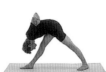

7 · Parsvottanasana (simple)

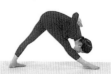

7 · Parsvottanasana (full pose)

9 · Uttanasana

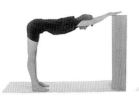

9 · Uttanasana
(on ledge)

14 · Sukhasana

15 · Virasana

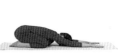

16 · Virasana
(forward bend)

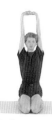

17 · Parvatasana
(in Virasana)

20 · Gomukhasana
(arms only)

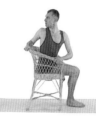

26 · Cross Bolsters

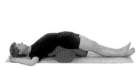

27 · Matsyasana (simple)

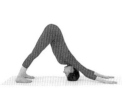

31 · Adho Mukha
Svanasana

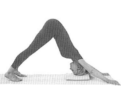

31 · Adho Mukha
Svanasana
(head supported)

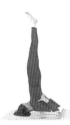

33 · Bharadvajasana
(on chair)

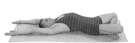

34 · Sarvangasana

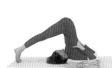

35 · Halasana

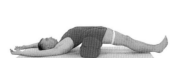

39 · Setu Bandha
Sarvangasana
(on bolster)

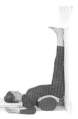

40 · Viparita Karani

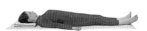

41 · Savasana

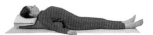

41 · Savasana
(on bolster)

WEEK 3

MONDAY, WEDNESDAY AND FRIDAY

31 · *Adho Mukha Svanasana*
9 · *Uttanasana*
  (on ledge)
1 · *Tadasana*
3 · *Trikonasana*
4 · *Parsvakonasana*
6 · *Virabhadrasana II*
*5 · *Virabhadrasana I*
9 · *Uttanasana*
*7 · *Parsvottanasana*
  (full pose)
33 · *Bharadvajasana*
  (on a chair)
14 · *Sukhasana*
17 · *Parvatasana*
  (in Sukhasana)
34 · *Sarvangasana*
35 · *Halasana*
41 · *Savasana*

TUESDAY AND THURSDAY

9 · *Uttanasana*
31 · *Adho Mukha Svanasana*
*18 · *Dandasana*
*22 · *Triang Mukhaikapada*
  Pascimottanasana
  (concave)
*24 · *Pascimottanasana*
  (concave)
36 · *Ardha Halasana*
*39 · *Setu Bandha*
  Sarvangasana
  (on bolster)
*30 · *Urdhva Prasarita*
  Padasana
41 · *Savasana*

SATURDAY

33 · *Bharadvajasana*
  (on a chair)
*32 · *Maricyasana*
  (standing)
1 · *Tadasana*
3 · *Trikonasana*
4 · *Parsvakonasana*
6 · *Virabhadrasana II*
5 · *Virabhadrasana I*
9 · *Uttanasana*
7 · *Parsvottanasana*
  (full pose)
*11 · *Garudasana*
15 · *Virasana*
17 · *Parvatasana*
  (in Virasana)
16 · *Virasana*
  (forward bend)
34 · *Sarvangasana*
35 · *Halasana*
41 · *Savasana*

SUNDAY

26 · *Cross Bolsters*
27 · *Matsyasana*
  (simple)
*28 · *Supta*
  Baddhakonasana
31 · *Adho Mukha*
  Svanasana
9 · *Uttanasana*
  (on ledge)
*38 · *Sarvangasana*
  (against wall)
36 · *Ardha Halasana*
39 · *Setu Bandha*
  Sarvangasana
  (on bolster)
40 · *Viparita Karani*
41 · *Savasana*
  (on bolster)

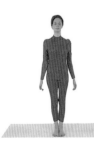

1 · *Tadasana*

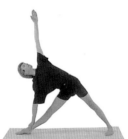

3 · *Trikonasana*

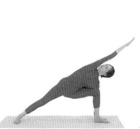

4 · *Parsvakonasana*

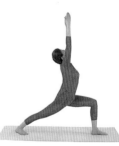

5 · *Virabhadrasana I*

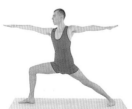

6 · *Virabhadrasana II*

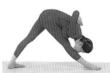

7 · *Parsvottanasana*
(full pose)

9 · *Uttanasana*

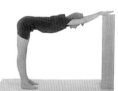

9 · *Uttanasana*
(on ledge)

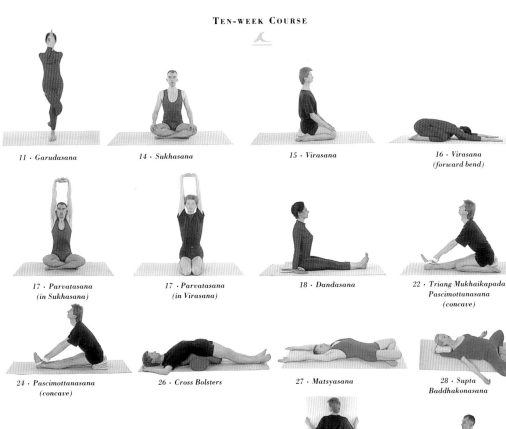

11 · Garudasana

14 · Sukhasana

15 · Virasana

16 · Virasana (forward bend)

17 · Parvatasana (in Sukhasana)

17 · Parvatasana (in Virasana)

18 · Dandasana

22 · Triang Mukhaikapada Pascimottanasana (concave)

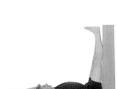

24 · Pascimottanasana (concave)

26 · Cross Bolsters

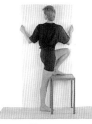

27 · Matsyasana

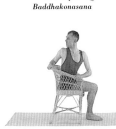

28 · Supta Baddhakonasana

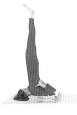

30 · Urdhva Prasarita Padasana

31 · Adho Mukha Svanasana

32 · Maricyasana (standing)

33 · Bharadvajasana (on chair)

34 · Sarvangasana

35 · Halasana

36 · Ardha Halasana

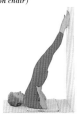

38 · Sarvangasana (against wall)

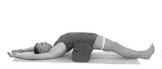

39 · Setu Bandha Sarvangasana (on bolster)

40 · Viparita Karani

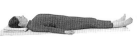

41 · Savasana

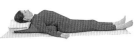

41 · Savasana (on bolster)

WEEK 4

MONDAY, WEDNESDAY AND FRIDAY	TUESDAY AND THURSDAY	SATURDAY	SUNDAY
15 · *Virasana*	32 · *Maricyasana (standing)*	1 · *Tadasana*	26 · *Cross Bolsters*
*13 · *Utthita Hasta Padangusthasana (forward and sideways)*	33 · *Bharadvajasana (on chair)*	2 · *Vrksasana*	27 · *Matsyasana (simple)*
1 · *Tadasana*	31 · *Adho Mukha Svanasana*	3 · *Trikonasana*	28 · *Supta Baddhakonasana*
3 · *Trikonasana*	18 · *Dandasana*	4 · *Parsvakonasana*	31 · *Adho Mukha Svanasana*
4 · *Parsvakonasana*	*21 · *Janusirsasana (concave)*	6 · *Virabhadrasana II*	9 · *Uttanasana (on ledge)*
6 · *Virabhadrasana II*	22 · *Triang Mukhaikapada Pascimottanasana (concave)*	5 · *Virabhadrasana I*	38 · *Sarvangasana (against wall)*
5 · *Virabhadrasana I*	*23 · *Maricyasana I (twist only)*	9 · *Uttanasana*	36 · *Ardha Halasana*
9 · *Uttanasana*	24 · *Pascimottanasana (concave)*	7 · *Parsvottanasana (full pose)*	39 · *Setu Bandha Sarvangasana (on bolster)*
7 · *Parsvottanasana (full pose)*	*25 · *Malasana (preparatory)*	11 · *Garudasana*	40 · *Viparita Karani*
17 · *Virasana (forward bend)*	34 · *Sarvangasana*	20 · *Gomukhasana (arms only)*	41 · *Savasana (on bolster)*
14 · *Sukhasana*	35 · *Halasana*	31 · *Adho Mukha Svanasana*	
27 · *Matsyasana*	41 · *Savasana*	34 · *Sarvangasana*	
34 · *Sarvangasana*		36 · *Ardha Halasana*	
35 · *Halasana*		41 · *Savasana*	
41 · *Savasana*			

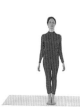

1 · Tadasana

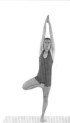

2 · Vrksasana

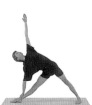

3 · Trikonasana

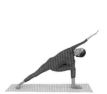

4 · Parsvakonasana

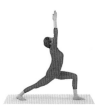

5 · Virabhadrasana I

6 · Virabhadrasana II

7 · Parsvottanasana

9 · Uttanasana

9 · Uttanasana (on ledge)

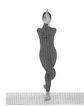

11 · Garudasana

Standing Poses
● Stretch legs up from ankle bones.
● In forward-facing poses, open the hips outward.
● Extend the front, sides and back of the body.

Sitting Poses
● Adjust the height of support in order not to slump in the lower back or push the lumber forward.
● In concave poses, lift and open the chest and move the back ribs in.

● In bent-legged poses, relax the groins and knees; take the thighs down without collapsing the back.
● In poses with straight legs, extend the legs and keep the thighs and knees down.

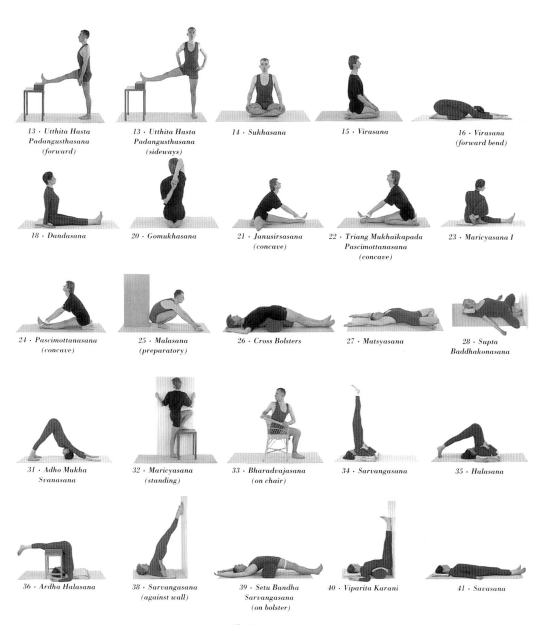

13 · Utthita Hasta
Padangusthasana
(forward)

13 · Utthita Hasta
Padangusthasana
(sideways)

14 · Sukhasana

15 · Virasana

16 · Virasana
(forward bend)

18 · Dandasana

20 · Gomukhasana

21 · Janusirsasana
(concave)

22 · Triang Mukhaikapada
Pascimottanasana
(concave)

23 · Maricyasana I

24 · Pascimottanasana
(concave)

25 · Malasana
(preparatory)

26 · Cross Bolsters

27 · Matsyasana

28 · Supta
Baddhakonasana

31 · Adho Mukha
Svanasana

32 · Maricyasana
(standing)

33 · Bharadvajasana
(on chair)

34 · Sarvangasana

35 · Halasana

36 · Ardha Halasana

38 · Sarvangasana
(against wall)

39 · Setu Bandha
Sarvangasana
(on bolster)

40 · Viparita Karani

41 · Savasana

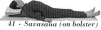

41 · Savasana (on bolster)

WEEK 5

Practise a mixture of dynamic and resting programmes from the previous four weeks.

WEEK 6

MONDAY, WEDNESDAY AND FRIDAY

1 · *Tadasana*
3 · *Trikonasana*
4 · *Parsvakonasana*
5 · *Virabhadrasana I*
9 · *Uttanasana*
6 · *Virabhadrasana II*
7 · *Parsvottanasana (full pose)*
*8 · *Prasarita Padottanasana*
16 · *Virasana (forward bend)*
34 · *Sarvangasana*
35 · *Halasana*
24 · *Pascimottanasana*
30 · *Urdhva Prasarita Padasana*
41 · *Savasana*

TUESDAY AND THURSDAY

9 · *Uttanasana*
31 · *Adho Mukha Svanasana*
*21 · *Janusirsasana (head supported)*
*22 · *Triang Mukhaikapada Pascimottanasana (head supported)*
*24 · *Pascimottanasana (head supported)*
23 · *Maricyasana I (twist only)*
34 · *Sarvangasana*
36 · *Ardha Halasana*
*39 · *Setu Bandha Sarvangasana (on bench)*
41 · *Savasana*

SATURDAY

13 · *Utthita Hasta Padangusthasana (forward and sideways)*
1 · *Tadasana*
3 · *Trikonasana*
4 · *Parsvakonasana*
5 · *Virabhadrasana I*
9 · *Uttanasana*
6 · *Virabhadrasana II*
7 · *Parsvottanasana (arms stretched)*
8 · *Prasarita Padottanasana*
*12 · *Utkatasana*
25 · *Malasana (preparatory)*
16 · *Virasana (forward bend)*
36 · *Ardha Halasana*
34 · *Sarvangasana*
41 · *Savasana*

SUNDAY

31 · *Adho Mukha Svanasana (head supported)*
16 · *Virasana (forward bend)*
9 · *Uttanasana*
30 · *Urdhva Prasarita Padasana*
27 · *Matsyasana (simple)*
28 · *Supta Baddhakonasana*
*37 · *Sarvangasana (on chair)*
36 · *Ardha Halasana*
41 · *Savasana (on bolster) (1) relaxing (2) observing the breath*

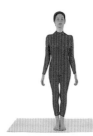

1 · Tadasana

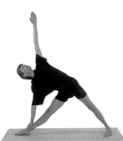

3 · Trikonasana

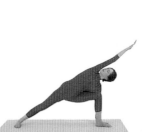

4 · Parsvakonasana

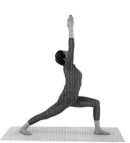

5 · Virabhadrasana I

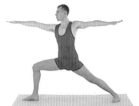

6 · Virabhadrasana II

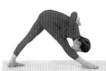

7 · Parsvottanasana (full pose)

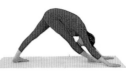

7 · Parsvottanasana (arms stretched)

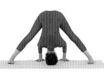

8 · Prasarita Padottanasana

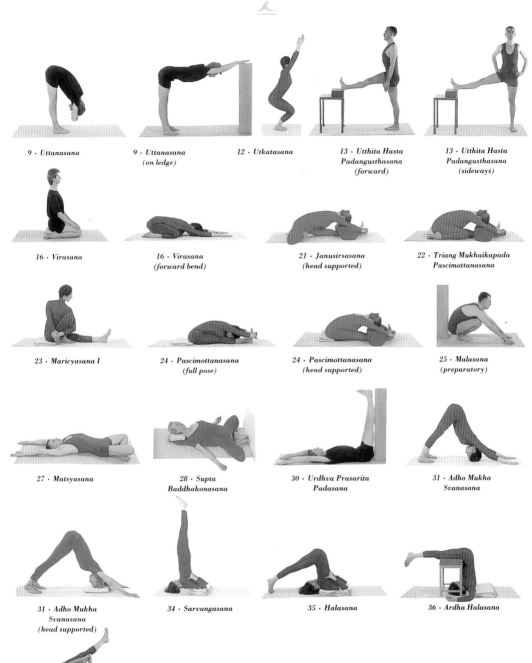

9 · *Uttanasana*

9 · *Uttanasana*
(on ledge)

12 · *Utkatasana*

13 · *Utthita Hasta*
Padangusthasana
(forward)

13 · *Utthita Hasta*
Padangusthasana
(sideways)

16 · *Virasana*

16 · *Virasana*
(forward bend)

21 · *Janusirsasana*
(head supported)

22 · *Triang Mukhaikapada*
Pascimottanasana

23 · *Maricyasana I*

24 · *Pascimottanasana*
(full pose)

24 · *Pascimottanasana*
(head supported)

25 · *Malasana*
(preparatory)

27 · *Matsyasana*

28 · *Supta*
Baddhakonasana

30 · *Urdhva Prasarita*
Padasana

31 · *Adho Mukha*
Svanasana

31 · *Adho Mukha*
Svanasana
(head supported)

34 · *Sarvangasana*

35 · *Halasana*

36 · *Ardha Halasana*

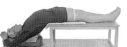

37 · *Sarvangasana*
(on chair)

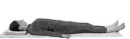

39 · *Setu Bandha*
Sarvangasana (on bench)

41 · *Savasana*

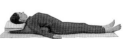

41 · *Savasana*
(on bolster)

WEEK 7

MONDAY, WEDNESDAY AND FRIDAY

15 · Virasana
31 · Adho Mukha Svanasana
1 · Tadasana
3 · Trikonasana
4 · Parsvakonasana
5 · Virabhadrasana I
9 · Uttanasana
6 · Virabhadrasana II
7 · Parsvottanasana
8 · Prasarita Padottanasana
16 · Virasana (forward bend)
*29 · Supta Virasana
28 · Supta Baddhakonasana
34 · Sarvangasana
35 · Halasana
24 · Pascimottanasana
41 · Savasana

TUESDAY AND THURSDAY

32 · Maricyasana (standing)
33 · Bharadvajasana (on chair)
9 · Uttanasana (on ledge)
31 · Adho Mukha Svanasana
14 · Sukhasana
17 · Parvatasana (in Sukhasana)
15 · Virasana
17 · Parvatasana (in Virasana)
18 · Dandasana
*19 · Siddhasana
20 · Gomukhasana (arms only)
* Namaste (in Virasana)
34 · Sarvangasana
35 · Halasana
41 · Savasana

SATURDAY

14 · Sukhasana
15 · Virasana
17 · Parvatasana (in Virasana)
31 · Adho Mukha Svanasana
18 · Dandasana
21 · Janusirsasana (concave)
22 · Triang Mukhaikapada Pascimottanasana (concave)
24 · Pascimottanasana (concave)
23 · Maricyasana I (twist only)
*33 · Bharadvajasana (preparatory)
25 · Malasana (preparatory)
34 · Sarvangasana
35 · Halasana
41 · Savasana

SUNDAY

31 · Adho Mukha Svanasana (head supported)
16 · Virasana (forward bend)
9 · Uttanasana
30 · Urdhva Prasarita Padasana
27 · Matsyasana (simple)
28 · Supta Baddhakonasana
37 · Sarvangasana (on chair)
36 · Ardha Halasana
41 · Savasana (on bolster)
(1) relaxing
(2) observing the breath

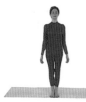

1 · Tadasana

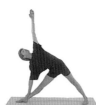

3 · Trikonasana

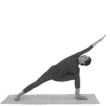

4 · Parsvakonasana

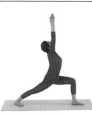

5 · Virabhadrasana I

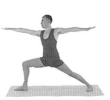

6 · Virabhadrasana II

7 · Parsvottanasana

8 · Prasarita Padottanasana

9 · Uttanasana

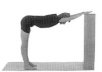

9 · Uttanasana (on ledge)

14 · Sukhasana

Sitting Poses
● In forward-bending poses, lengthen the whole trunk.
● Look up without compressing the back of the neck.

● Extend the upper arms away from the shoulders, the forearms away from the elbows, and the hands away from the wrists.
● Catch further and further.

Twists
● Keep the legs stable as you turn.
● Move the whole trunk when turning. ● Catch further. ● Turn the head without tensing the neck.

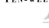

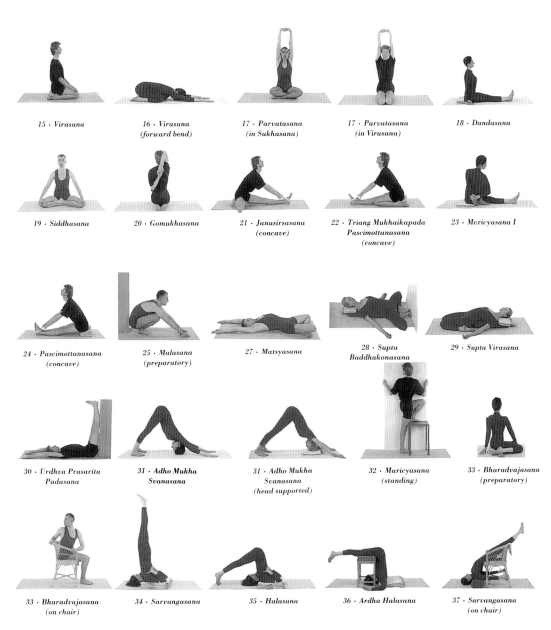

15 · *Virasana*

16 · *Virasana*
(forward bend)

17 · *Parvatasana*
(in Sukhasana)

17 · *Parvatasana*
(in Virasana)

18 · *Dandasana*

19 · *Siddhasana*

20 · *Gomukhasana*

21 · *Janusirsasana*
(concave)

22 · *Triang Mukhaikapada*
Pascimottanasana
(concave)

23 · *Maricyasana I*

24 · *Pascimottanasana*
(concave)

25 · *Malasana*
(preparatory)

27 · *Matsyasana*

28 · *Supta*
Baddhakonasana

29 · *Supta Virasana*

30 · *Urdhva Prasarita*
Padasana

31 · **Adho Mukha**
Svanasana

31 · *Adho Mukha*
Svanasana
(head supported)

32 · *Maricyasana*
(standing)

33 · *Bharadvajasana*
(preparatory)

33 · *Bharadvajasana*
(on chair)

34 · *Sarvangasana*

35 · *Halasana*

36 · *Ardha Halasana*

37 · *Sarvangasana*
(on chair)

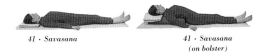

41 · *Savasana*

41 · *Savasana*
(on bolster)

WEEK 8

MONDAY, WEDNESDAY AND FRIDAY	TUESDAY AND THURSDAY	SATURDAY	SUNDAY
1 · Tadasana	9 · Uttanasana (on ledge)	33 · Bharadvajasana (on chair)	26 · Cross Bolsters
2 · Vrksasana	31 · Adho Mukha Svanasana	32 · Maricyasana (standing)	27 · Matsyasana
3 · Trikonasana	16 · Virasana (forward bend)	1 · Tadasana	28 · Supta Baddhakonasana
4 · Parsvakonasana	18 · Dandasana	3 · Trikonasana	29 · Supta Virasana
5 · Virabhadrasana I	*21 · Janusirsasana (full pose)	4 · Parsvakonasana	16 · Virasana (forward bend)
9 · Uttanasana	*22 · Triang Mukhaikapada Pascimottanasana (full pose)	5 · Virabhadrasana I	9 · Uttanasana
6 · Virabhadrasana II	*24 · Pascimottanasana (full pose)	9 · Uttanasana	31 · Adho Mukha Svanasana
7 · Parsvottanasana (full pose)	33 · Bharadvajasana (preparatory)	6 · Virabhadrasana II	37 · Sarvangasana (on chair)
9 · Uttanasana	36 · Ardha Halasana	7 · Parsvottanasana (arms stretched)	36 · Ardha Halasana
*10 · Padangusthasana	39 · Setu Bandha Sarvangasana (on bench)	8 · Prasarita Padottanasana	39 · Setu Bandha Sarvangasana (on bench)
12 · Utkatasana	40 · Viparita Karani	25 · Malasana (preparatory)	41 · Savasana (on bolster) (1) relaxing (2) observing the breath (3) lengthening the breath
11 · Garudasana	41 · Savasana	31 · Adho Mukha Svanasana	
16 · Virasana (forward bend)		16 · Virasana (forward bend)	
36 · Ardha Halasana		34 · Sarvangasana	
41 · Savasana		35 · Halasana	
		41 · Savasana	

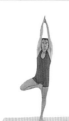

1 · Tadasana

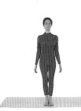

2 · Vrksasana

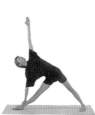

3 · Trikonasana

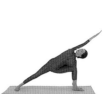

4 · Parsvakonasana

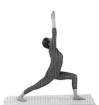

5 · Virabhadrasana I

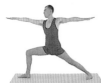

6 · Virabhadrasana II

7 · Parsvottanasana

7 · Parsvottanasana (arms stretched)

8 · Prasarita Padottanasana

9 · Uttanasana

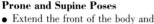
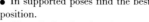

Prone and Supine Poses
● Extend the front of the body and keep it relaxed; enjoy opening the chest; breathe evenly.

● In supported poses find the best position.
● Place the head and neck in a comfortable position.

Inverted Poses
● In supported poses, experiment with the height of the support to make it most effective.

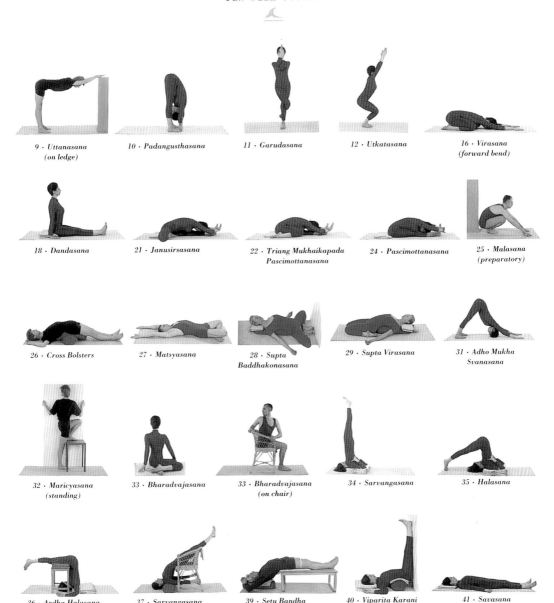

9 · Uttanasana
(on ledge)

10 · Padangusthasana

11 · Garudasana

12 · Utkatasana

16 · Virasana
(forward bend)

18 · Dandasana

21 · Janusirsasana

22 · Triang Mukhaikapada
Pascimottanasana

24 · Pascimottanasana

25 · Malasana
(preparatory)

26 · Cross Bolsters

27 · Matsyasana

28 · Supta
Baddhakonasana

29 · Supta Virasana

31 · Adho Mukha
Svanasana

32 · Maricyasana
(standing)

33 · Bharadvajasana

33 · Bharadvajasana
(on chair)

34 · Sarvangasana

35 · Halasana

36 · Ardha Halasana

37 · Sarvangasana
(on chair)

39 · Setu Bandha
Sarvangasana
(on bench)

40 · Viparita Karani

41 · Savasana

41 · Savasana
(on bolster)

- Keep the chest open and lifted while remaining relaxed.
- Keep the head in line with the rest of the body.

- Extend the neck without tension.
- Adjust the arms and shoulders to make them even, and get in a comfortable position.

Relaxation
- Place yourself accurately.
- Breathe quietly.
- Relax, letting go completely.

WEEK 9

MONDAY, WEDNESDAY AND FRIDAY

13 · Utthita Hasta Padangusthasana (forward and sideways)
1 · Tadasana
3 · Trikonasana
4 · Parsvakonasana
5 · Virabhadrasana I
9 · Uttanasana
6 · Virabhadrasana II
7 · Parsvottanasana
8 · Prasarita Padottanasana
10 · Padangusthasana
31 · Adho Mukha Svanasana
16 · Virasana (forward bend)
34 · Sarvangasana
21 · Janusirsasana
24 · Pascimottanasana
41 · Savasana

TUESDAY AND THURSDAY

15 · Virasana
17 · Parvatasana (in Virasana)
14 · Sukhasana
17 · Parvatasana (in Sukhasana)
20 · Gomukhasana (arms only)
33 · Bharadvajasana (on chair)
32 · Maricyasana (standing)
18 · Dandasana
23 · Maricyasana I (twist only)
*33 · Bharadvajasana
25 · Malasana
34 · Sarvangasana
35 · Halasana
24 · Pascimottanasana
41 · Savasana

SATURDAY

1 · Tadasana
2 · Vrksasana
11 · Garudasana
12 · Utkatasana
15 · Virasana
19 · Siddhasana
18 · Dandasana
21 · Janusirsasana
22 · Triang Mukhaikapada Pascimottanasana
24 · Pascimottanasana
31 · Adho Mukha Svanasana
34 · Sarvangasana
35 · Halasana
41 · Savasana

SUNDAY

26 · Cross Bolsters
27 · Matsyasana
28 · Supta Baddhakonasana
29 · Supta Virasana
16 · Virasana (forward bend)
9 · Uttanasana
31 · Adho Mukha Svanasana
37 · Sarvangasana (on chair)
36 · Ardha Halasana
39 · Setu Bandha Sarvangasana (on bench)
41 · Savasana (on bolster)
   (1) relaxing
   (2) observing the breath
   (3) lengthening the breath

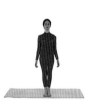

1 · Tadasana

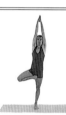

2 · Vrksasana

3 · Trikonasana

4 · Parsvakonasana

5 · Virabhadrasana I

6 · Virabhadrasana II

7 · Parsvottanasana

8 · Prasarita Padottanasana

9 · Uttanasana

10 · Padangusthasana

11 · Garudasana

12 · Utkatasana

13 · Utthita Hasta Padangusthasana (forward)

13 · Utthita Hasta Padangusthasana (sideways)

14 · Sukhasana

15 · Virasana

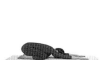

16 · Virasana
(forward bend)

17 · Parvatasana
(in Sukhasana)

17 · Parvatasana
(in Virasana)

18 · Dandasana

19 · Siddhasana

20 · Gomukhasana
(arms only)

21 · Janusirsasana

22 · Triang Mukhaikapada
Pascimottanasana

23 · Maricyasana I

24 · Pascimottanasana

25 · Malasana
(preparatory)

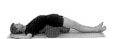

26 · Cross Bolsters

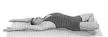

27 · Matsyasana

28 · Supta
Baddhakonasana

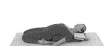

29 · Supta
Virasana

31 · Adho Mukha
Svanasana

32 · Maricyasana
(standing)

33 · Bharadvajasana

33 · Bharadvajasana
(on chair)

34 · Sarvangasana

35 · Halasana

36 · Ardha Halasana

37 · Sarvangasana
(on chair)

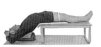

39 · Setu Bandha
Sarvangasana

41 · Savasana

41 · Savasana (on bolster)

WEEK 10

Practise any programmes from weeks 6-9 inclusive.

ASANAS FOR MENSTRUATION

Although menstruation is a normal and natural process, it involves physiological and metabolic changes, and yoga practice takes account of the altered condition of the body at this time. The postures given in this programme are a combination of restful ones and those that ease pain and strain.

Strenuous postures such as standing and inverted poses, and vigorous extensions in any poses, should be avoided. Yoga practice generally helps complaints associated with the menstrual cycle, such as cramp, irregularity, scanty or excessive bleeding, backache and pre-menstrual tension.

SUPTA VIRASANA
HERO POSE (SUPINE)

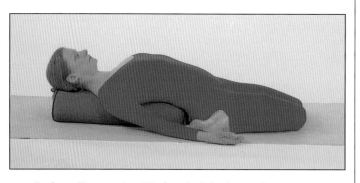

Do Supta Virasana (no. 29). Stay for 3–5 minutes, then come up.

SUPTA BADDHAKONASANA
SUPINE COBBLER POSE

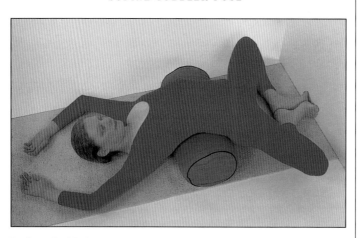

Do Supta Baddhakonasana (no. 28) with a crosswise bolster under the waist. Stay for 5–8 minutes, then come up.

BADDHAKONASANA
COBBLER POSE

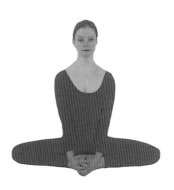

Sit in Dandasana (no. 18) against a wall, on one or two folded blankets. Bend the knees to the sides. Bring the feet together and line them up, with the soles touching. Bring the heels as close as possible to the pubis. Hold the toes. If you are sitting too high to reach them, hold the ankles. Stretch the thighs toward the knees and take the knees down. Stretch the trunk up and open the chest. Keep the head level.

Stay for 3–5 minutes, then release.

UPAVISTAKONASANA
WIDE-ANGLED SEATED POSE

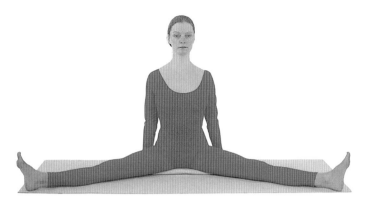

Sit in Dandasana (no. 18) on one or two folded blankets, with the back against a wall. Spread the legs apart, as wide as possible. Keep the front of the legs facing the ceiling and the feet upright. Straighten the knees and pull the thigh muscles back towards the groin. Draw the trunk up, extend the spine up and open the chest. Breathe evenly. Stay for 2–3 minutes, then release.

JANUSIRSASANA
HEAD TO KNEE POSE

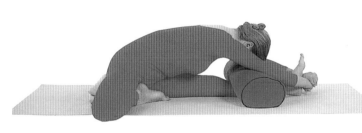

Do Janusirsasana (no. 21), variant with head supported.
   Stay for 1–2 minutes, then repeat on the other side.

TRIANG MUKHAIKAPADA PASCIMOTTANASANA
FORWARD BEND WITH LEG BENT BACK

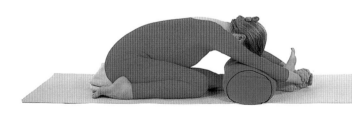

Do Triang Mukhaikapada Pascimottanasana (no. 22).
   Stay for 1–2 minutes, then repeat on the other side.

- If you experience cramp during menstruation, do the forward bends with the back concave.
- If you are stiff, rest the head on a stool.
- If there is strain in the knees, support it and reduce the length of time in the posture.

ARDHA BADDHA PADMA PASCIMOTTANASANA
HALF-LOTUS FORWARD BEND

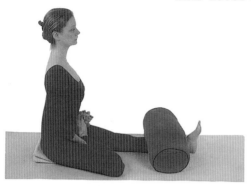

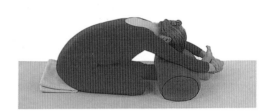

1 *Sit in Dandasana (no. 18). Bend the right leg and place the foot on top of the left thigh, in the groin. Place a bolster on the left shin.*

2 *Bend forward, hold the left foot and rest the head on the bolster. Stay for 30–40 seconds, then repeat on the other side.*

● *If there is strain in the knee, support it on a rolled blanket. Do not tense the knee.*

MARICYASANA I
SIMPLE TWIST WITH FORWARD BEND

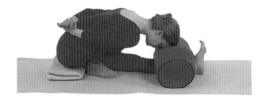

Do Maricyasana I (no. 23). Turn the trunk forward and bend down over the straight leg. Rest the head on the bolster. Keep the abdomen soft. Stay for 30–40 seconds, then repeat on the other side.

PASCIMOTTANASANA
FULL FORWARD BEND WITH HEAD SUPPORTED

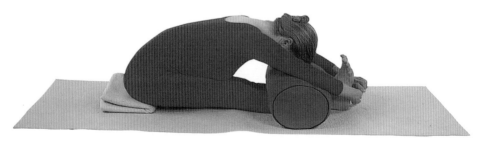

Do Pascimottanasana (no. 24) resting the head on a bolster. Stay for 2–3 minutes, then come up.

SETU BANDHA SARVANGASANA
NECK BALANCE BACK ARCH

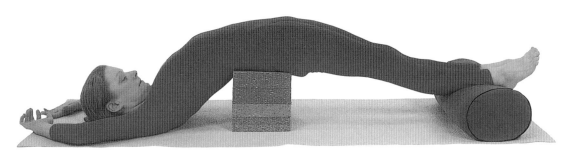

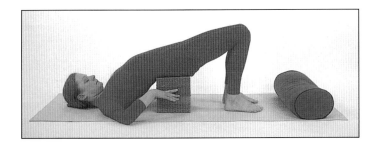

1 *Above: Do Setu Bandha Sarvangasana (no. 39). Lie over a support, such as a bench, folded blankets or bolsters. Stay for 5–8 minutes.*

2 *Left: To come down, bend the knees and hold the bench, blankets or bolsters. Slide back, then turn to the side and get up.*

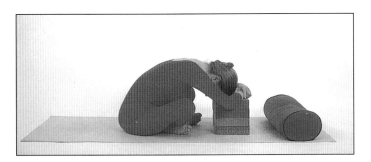

3 *Sit and bend forward, resting your head on the support. If the lower back pulls, take the buttocks a little further back, or sit on a bolster and bend down.*

SAVASANA
CORPSE POSE

Do Savasana (no. 41) for 5–10 minutes, then turn to the side and come up.

ASANAS FOR HEADACHES

The sequence of postures given here is designed to alleviate headaches caused by stress and tension.

The bandage, which we show wound round the head for the forward bends, can be used from the beginning. It relieves the internal pressure that comes with headaches. Care should be taken not to tie a bandage too tightly.

As you become stronger through regular yoga practice, you should find that you suffer less from headaches, and can get rid of them more easily.

CROSS BOLSTERS

Lie over Cross Bolsters (no. 26).

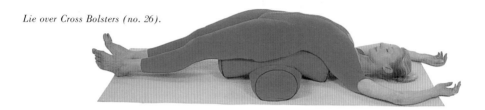

SUPTA VIRASANA
RECLINING HERO POSE

Do Supta Virasana (no. 29).

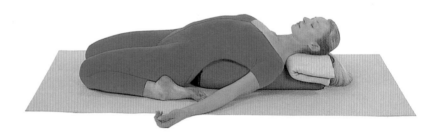

SUPTA BADDHAKONASANA
SUPINE COBBLER POSE

Do Supta Baddhakonasana (no. 28).

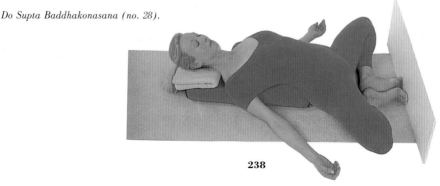

USING A BANDAGE

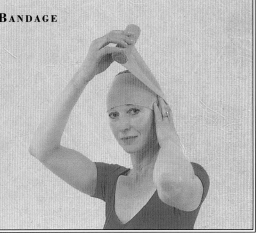

A firmly tied bandage round the head is very soothing for headaches. It cools the eyes, temples and head.

Wind a bandage several times round the forehead and back of the skull. Pull the bandage firmly but do not make it too tight.

If you have eyestrain also cover the eyes: in this case wind the bandage lightly two or three times round the eyes at the beginning.

UTTANASANA
— STANDING BEND (HEAD SUPPORTED) —

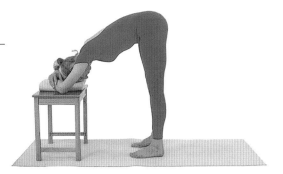

Do Uttanasana (no. 9) as follows: place a folded blanket on a stool. Stand with the feet 12–18 inches (30–45 cm) apart in front of the stool. Bend down and rest the head on it. Fold the arms and relax.

Stay for 1–2 minutes, then come up.

ADHO MUKHA SVANASANA
—— DOG POSE (HEAD SUPPORTED) ——

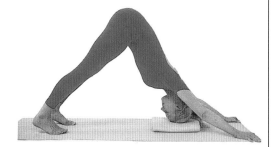

Do Adho Mukha Svanasana (no. 31), variant with head supported.

JANUSIRSASANA
HEAD-TO-KNEE POSE (HEAD SUPPORTED)

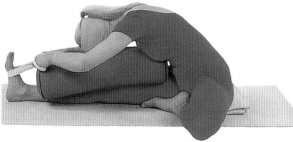

Do Janusirsasana (no. 21), variant with head on bolster, with the head bandaged. Place a bolster lengthwise on the extended leg and rest the head on it. If it is difficult to hold the foot, use a belt. Relax.

Stay for 2–5 minutes, then repeat on the other side.

PASCIMOTTANASANA
FULL FORWARD BEND (HEAD SUPPORTED)

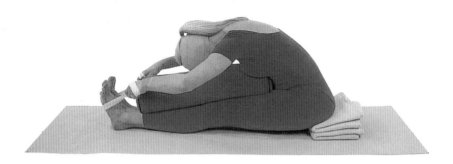

Do Pascimottanasana (no. 24) with the head bandaged. Place a bolster lengthwise on the legs and rest the head on it. Hold the feet with the hands or with a belt. Relax. Stay for 3–5 minutes,

ARDHA HALASANA
HALF-PLOUGH POSE

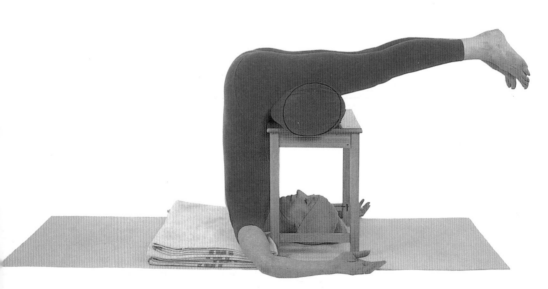

Do Ardha Halasana (no. 36). Stay for 5–8 minutes. To come down, bring the legs back a little, push the stool away and carefully slide down.

SETU BANDHA SARVANGASANA
NECK BALANCE WITH BACK ARCH

Do Setu Bandha Sarvangasana
(no. 39), using two bolsters or a
pile of blankets under the lower
back. Support the legs if necessary.
Relax.
 Stay for 5–8 minutes, then come
down.

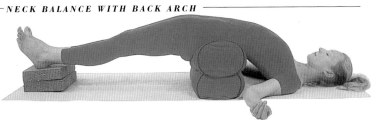

VIPARITA KARANI
RESTFUL INVERSION

Do Viparita Karani (no. 40). Stay
for 5–8 minutes. Bend the knees,
slide backward, turn to the side
and get up.

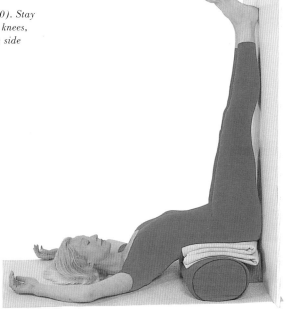

SAVASANA
CORPSE POSE

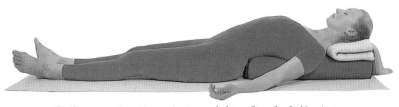

Do Savasana (no. 41), variant on a bolster. Stay for 5–10 minutes.

ASANAS FOR STIFF NECK AND SHOULDERS

The postures given here are designed to relieve stiffness and pain in the neck and shoulders. These problems are extremely common as well as troublesome; they are often caused by poor posture or life-style stress.

The postures emphasize freeing and stretching the affected areas to increase mobility. With time and regular practice, the neck and shoulders will become stronger and more supple, and will move to a more anatomically correct position. Gradually, pain and discomfort should diminish.

All the postures can be attempted by beginners.

TRIKONASANA
TRIANGLE POSE

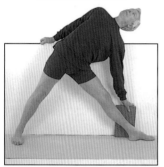

Do Trikonasana (no. 3) standing against a ledge or wall. Place one hand on a block and grip the ledge with the other hand to turn the trunk more. Stay for 20–30 seconds, then repeat on the other side.

PARSVAKONASANA
LATERAL ANGLE POSE

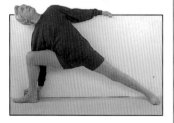

Do Parsvakonasana (no. 4), standing against a ledge or wall. Place the right hand on a block and grip the ledge with the left hand. Turn the trunk with the help of the hands. Stay for 20–30 seconds, then repeat on the other side.

ARDHA CANDRASANA
HALF-MOON POSE

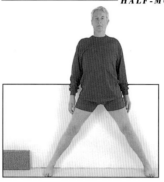

1 *Stand with your back 3–6 inches (7.5–15 cm) away from a ledge or wall. Take the feet 3¹⁄₂– 4 ft (105–120 cm) apart. Place a block against the wall, about 12 inches (30 cm) from the right foot.*

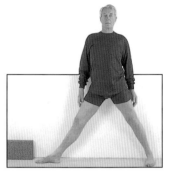

2 *Turn the left foot 15° in and the right foot 90° out.*

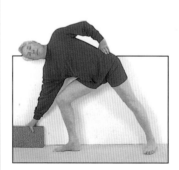

3 *Bend the right knee, lean sideways to the right and place the right hand on the block. Bring the left foot slightly in, toward the right foot. Hold the ledge.*

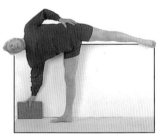

4 *Bring your weight onto the right foot and hand. At the same time, straighten the right leg and place the left foot on the ledge. Tighten both knees. Place the left hand on the left hip and turn the trunk forward. Keep the back against the wall. Stay for 20–30 seconds.*

To come down, bend the right leg and lower the left leg to the floor. Repeat on the other side.

VIRASANA FORWARD BEND

HERO POSE

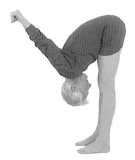

Do Virasana Forward Bend (no. 16). Place a bolster or folded blankets on the heels.

UTTANASANA WITH A POLE

STANDING FORWARD BEND

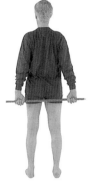

1 Stand with the feet hip-width apart. Hold a pole or stick horizontally behind the back, with the palms facing up.

2 Bend forward and raise the pole up and over, as far as you can. Keep the elbows straight. Do not bend the knees. Stay for 10–20 seconds, then come up.

URDHVA MUKHA SVANASANA

DOG POSE HEAD UP (ON CHAIR)

Place a sturdy stool or chair against a wall. Grip the edges firmly with the hands. Bend the legs and rest the tops of the thighs on the seat. Step back and straighten the legs. Keep the arms firm, roll the shoulders back and stretch the trunk up. Curve the back and look up. Do not hold the breath. Stay for 15–20 seconds, then come down.

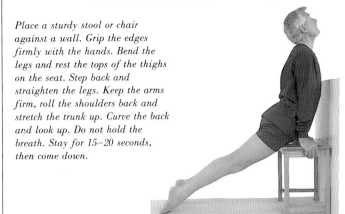

ADHO MUKHA SVANASANA

DOG POSE HEAD DOWN

Do Adho Mukha Svanasana (no. 31). Stretch the arms up strongly and lift the shoulders and trunk. Stay for 20–30 seconds, then come down.

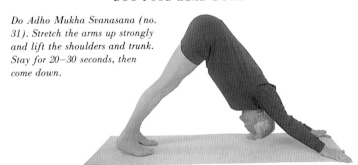

PARVATASANA IN VIRASANA

MOUNTAIN POSE

Do Parvatasana (no. 17), sitting in Virasana (no. 15). Stay for 20–30 seconds, then change the interlock of the fingers.

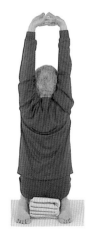

GOMUKHASANA
(ARMS ONLY)
— HEAD OF COW POSE —

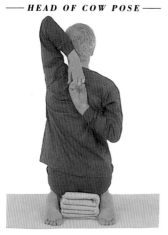

Sit in Virasana (no. 15). Catch the hands in Gomukhasana (no. 20). Stay for 20–30 seconds, then repeat on the other side.

NAMASTE
(IN VIRASANA)
— PRAYER POSITION —

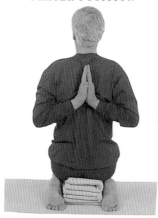

Sit in Virasana (no. 15) and join the palms behind the back in Namaste (no. 7). Stay for 30–60 seconds, then release. If the wrists hurt do not shake them but allow them to come to normal slowly.

BHARADVAJASANA
— SIMPLE TWIST —

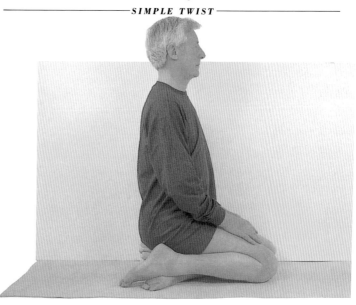

1 *Do Bharadvajasana (no. 33) sitting on one or two folded* *blankets near a wall or ledge. Line yourself up.*

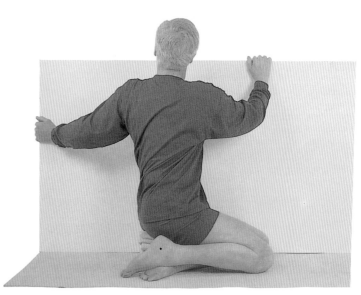

2 *Turn toward the ledge, gripping it with both hands to help you turn as far as you can.* *Turn the shoulders and chest. Stay for 20–30 seconds, then repeat on the other side.*

MARICYASANA III

—————— *TWIST WITH OPPOSITE ARM AGAINST LEG* ——————

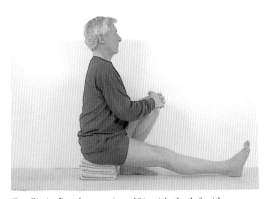 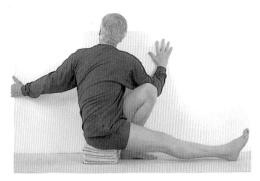

1 *Sit in Dandasana (no. 18) with the left side against a wall or ledge. Bend the left leg up and bring the foot close to its own thigh. Hold the knee and stretch the trunk up.*

2 *Turn the trunk toward the wall. Bring the right elbow to the outer edge of the left knee, fix the upper arm firmly against the knee and hold the ledge. Use the hands to help you turn as far as you can. Stay for 20–30 seconds, then repeat on the other side.*

SETU BANDHA SARVANGASANA

—————— *NECK BALANCE BACK ARCH* ——————

Do Setu Bandha Sarvangasana (no. 39), variant on bench.

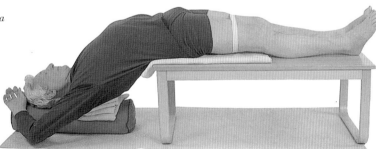

SAVASANA

—————— *CORPSE POSE* ——————

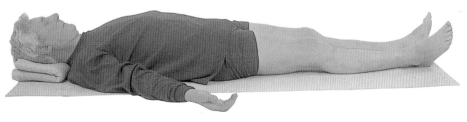

Do Savasana (no. 41). Stay for 5–10 minutes, then turn to the side and get up.

ASANAS FOR BACKACHE

The postures given in this programme are designed to alleviate simple backaches, both of the lower and the upper back. They are not, however, intended for severe conditions such as slipped disc or pain resulting from a fracture or other medical problem; in these cases advice should be sought from a teacher experienced in yoga therapy.

The postures are all suitable for beginners. With continued practice, back problems should decrease and may disappear altogether. The back should become stronger and less liable to ache.

When doing the postures, do not jerk or move suddenly. Keep the affected part passive and move below or above it. Do not focus on the painful part directly. In the beginning, the painful part needs to be rested, not worked.

HALF UTTANASANA
— HALF FORWARD BEND —

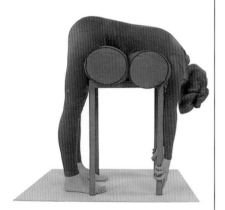

Stand in front of a tall stool or small table. Place neatly folded blankets or bolsters on it to raise the height to that of your hips. Take the feet about hip-width apart. Stand on tip-toe and bend over the stool, tucking the edge of the blankets or bolster into the groin. Extend the abdomen and the front ribs over the bolster. Then stretch the heels to touch the ground. Relax the arms down, or hold the legs of the stool. Keep the legs vertical. Allow the spine and back ribs to relax.

Stay for 30–60 seconds. Come up carefully.

BHARADVAJASANA ON CHAIR
CHAIR TWIST

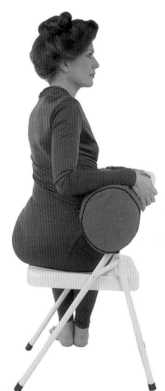

Sit sideways on a chair. Stretch the trunk up. Take one or two breaths. Turn toward the back of the chair. Place a bolster or folded blankets between the back of the chair and the abdomen. Grip the back of the chair and turn as far as possible. Do not hold the breath.

Stay for 20–30 seconds, then repeat on the other side.

FORWARD BEND

Sit on the chair and spread the legs apart. Place a bolster or folded blanket across the thighs, tucking it into the groin. Extend the abdomen and the front ribs over it. Bend down. Take the arms inside the legs of the chair and hold the back legs of the chair. Relax the head.

Stay for 20–30 seconds. Come up carefully, without jerking.

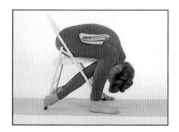

MARICYASANA (STANDING)
STANDING TWIST

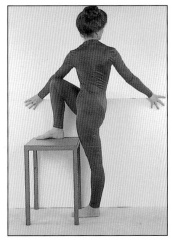

Do Maricyasana (standing) (no. 32). Stay for 20–30 seconds, then repeat on the other side.

PARSVA PAVANA MUKTASANA
WIND RELEASING POSE

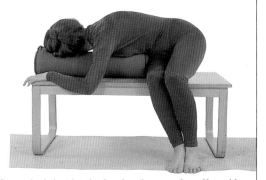

Sit at the left side of a low bench or sturdy coffee table. Place a bolster or folded blankets lengthwise on top of it, to your right. Turn toward the bolster. Bend down and rest the length of the front of the body along it. Hold the bench or bolster and turn the head to the right. Keep the legs facing forward as much as possible. Extend the front ribs and relax the back.

Stay for 30–60 seconds, then repeat on the other side. After bending to the sides, do Pavana Muktasana: sit at the front of the bench, spread the knees apart and bend down. If bending is easy, it is a sign of recovery.

UTTHITA TRIKONASANA
EXTENDED TRIANGLE POSE

Do Trikonasana (no. 3) with the back against a wall. If possible, find a wall with a projecting corner so that you can hold it.

Stay for 20–30 seconds, then repeat on the other side.

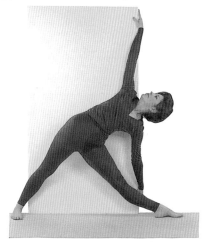

ARDHA CANDRASANA
HALF-MOON POSE

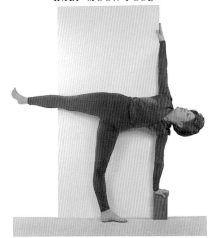

Do Ardha Candrasana against the wall (see "Asanas for Stiff Hips"). Hold on to a projecting corner of a wall with the top hand. Place the lower hand on a block and the raised heel on the wall. Turn the trunk upward.

Stay for 20–30 seconds, then repeat on the other side.

● *If you have sciatica, turn the front foot out 120°.*

PARSVOTTANASANA
— SIDEWAYS STRETCH —

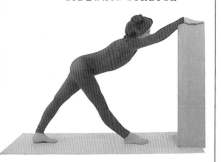

Do Parsvottanasana (no. 7) as follows: stand in Tadasana (no. 1) about 3 ft (90 cm) from a ledge with your right side facing it. Take the feet 3½–4 ft (105–120 cm) apart. Turn the left foot 45°–60° in and the right foot 90° out. Turn the trunk to face the ledge. Bring the left hip forward in line with the right. Bend down and place the hands on the ledge. Straighten the arms. Keep the hips level and the legs straight. Stretch the trunk.

Stay for 20–30 seconds, then repeat on the other side.

UTTANASANA
FORWARD EXTENSION
— ON LEDGE —

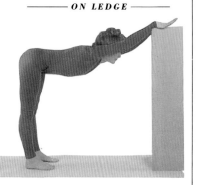

Do Uttanasana (variant on ledge) (no. 9). Stay for 20–30 seconds, then come up.

ADHO MUKHA SVANASANA
— DOG POSE HEAD DOWN —

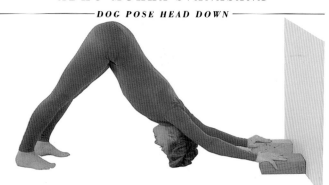

Do Adho Mukha Svanasana (no. 31) as follows: place two blocks against a wall about 18 inches (45 cm) or shoulder-width apart. Kneel down and place the hands on the blocks. Raise the hips and straighten the arms and legs to make an inverted "V" shape. If necessary, walk the feet further back. Keep the hips up. Stretch the arms and trunk up, away from the blocks. Relax the head.

Stay for 20–30 seconds, then come down.

VIRASANA FORWARD BEND
— HERO POSE —

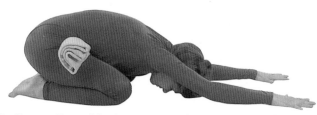

Do Virasana Forward Bend (no. 16) as follows: place a rolled or folded blanket on the thighs and tuck it into the groin. Extend the abdomen over it.

Stay for 30–60 seconds.

SUKHASANA (WITH SIDEWAYS BEND)
— EASY POSE —

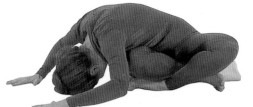

Sit in Sukhasana (no. 14) with the legs crossed simply. Turn to the right and bend down over the right leg. Stay for 30–60 seconds, then change the cross legs and bend to the right.

ARDHA HALASANA
HALF-PLOUGH POSE

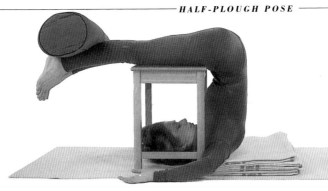

Do Ardha Halasana (no. 36). If possible, ask someone to place a weight such as a bolster or pile of blankets on the lower calves.

Stay for 5–8 minutes, then remove the bolster and slide down.

SUPTA PADANGUSTHASANA
RECLINING FINGER-TO-FOOT POSE

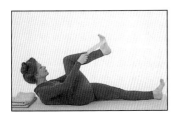

1 Lie on the floor in a straight line. If necessary, place a blanket under the head. Bend the right leg over the abdomen and place a belt round the foot.

2 Hold the belt with both hands and straighten the right leg up. Press the left thigh down. Stretch the left leg along the floor and the right leg up.

Stay for 20–30 seconds, then bend the right leg and bring it down. Line yourself up again and repeat on the other side.

VARIANT

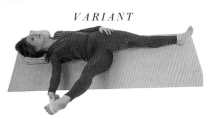

Lie in a straight line. Follow the method given in steps 1 and 2.

Press the left thigh down with the left hand. Raise and straighten the right leg, then turn it outward and take it down to the right. Keep both legs stretched.

Stay for 20–30 seconds. Raise the leg, bend it and lower it to the floor. Repeat on the other side.

SAVASANA
CORPSE POSE

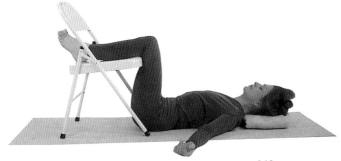

Do Savasana (no. 41) as follows: bend the legs and rest the calves on a stool or chair. Relax.

Stay for 5–10 minutes. Bring the legs down, turn to the side and get up carefully.

ASANAS FOR STIFF HIPS

The sequence of postures in this programme is designed to make the hips and lower back work more efficiently, by increasing mobility and strength. Too often the hip and sacro-iliac joints become stiff through incorrect use, or under- or over use. Often they become affected by arthritic conditions. Ease of movement of these joints is important, especially in later life when ordinary movements, such as sitting, standing and walking, may become slow and difficult. Yoga postures are an invaluable tool to prevent this.

BHARADVAJASANA (ON CHAIR)
CHAIR TWIST

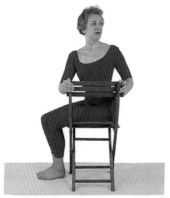

Do Bharadvajasana (no. 33) variant on a chair. Stay for 20–30 seconds, then repeat on the other side.

MARICYASANA (STANDING)

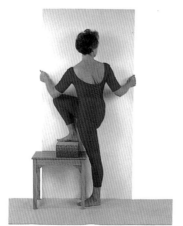

Do Maricyasana (standing) (no. 32).

UTTHITA TRIKONASANA
TRIANGLE POSE

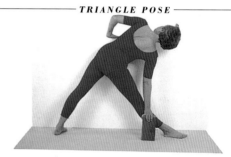

Do Trikonasana (no. 3), facing a wall or ledge. Place a block by the outer edge of the right foot and put your hand on it. Grip the wall or ledge with the left hand. Use the hands to help you to turn the trunk toward the wall and press the right hip forward. Stay for 20–30 seconds, then repeat on the other side.

UTTHITA PARSVAKONASANA
LATERAL ANGLE POSE

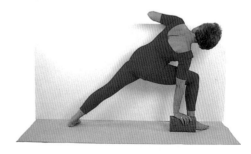

Do Parsvakonasana (no. 4) facing a wall or ledge. Place a block on the floor by the right foot and place your hand on it. With the left hand, grip the ledge or press the wall. Lift the right hip and press it toward the wall. Turn the trunk toward the wall, with the hands. Stay for 20–30 seconds, then repeat on the other side.

VIRABHADRASANA I
WARRIOR POSE I

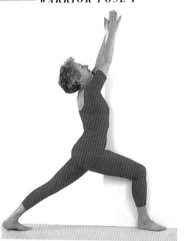

PARIVRTTA TRIKONASANA
REVERSE TRIANGLE POSE

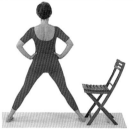

Do Virabhadrasana I (no. 5) as follows: stand sideways in a doorway facing the door post (or face a column). Hold it and take the right leg forward along the wall, with the inner thigh touching the door post. Bend the knee to a right angle. Step back with the left leg and straighten it. If necessary, raise the heel. Turn the hips and pelvis toward the post and stretch the front of the body up against it. Press the lower back (sacrum) toward the post, without raising the right hip. Take the hands higher to gain the maximum stretch. Stay for 20–30 seconds, then repeat on the other side.

1 *Stand in Tadasana (no. 1) with a chair placed about 3 ft (105 cm) to your right. Place the hands on the hips and spread the legs 3½–4 ft (90–120 cm) apart.*

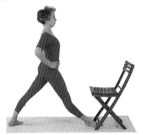

2 *Turn the left foot 45–60° in and the right foot 90° out. Turn the hips and trunk to the right.*

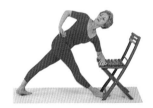

VIRABHADRASANA II
WARRIOR POSE II

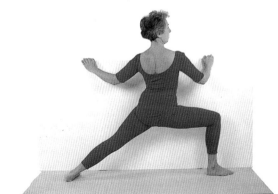

Do Virabhadrasana II (no. 6) facing a wall or a ledge. Hold the ledge firmly. Press the right hip toward the wall and move the right knee away from it. Stay for 20–30 seconds. Repeat on the other side.

3 *Revolve the trunk further and take it down toward the chair, so that the left side faces the floor and the right side faces the ceiling. Rest the left forearm on the seat of the chair and grip the edge. Keep the right hand on the hip. Extend the trunk and turn the hips and trunk as far as you can. Stay for 20–30 seconds, then repeat on the other side.*

UTTHITA HASTA PADANGUSTHASANA
EXTENDED LEG RAISING
All three variants should be practised.

FORWARD

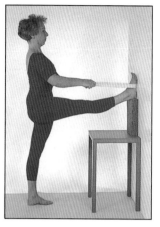

SIDEWAYS

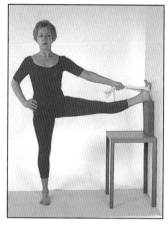

TWIST

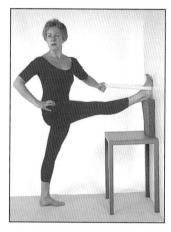

Place a high stool against a wall. Do Utthita Hasta Padangusthasana (no. 13) forward, using a belt to hold the raised foot. Stretch the trunk up. Stay for 30–60 seconds, then repeat on the other side.

Place a high stool against a wall. Do Utthita Hasta Padangusthasana (no. 13) sideways, using a belt to hold the raised foot. Stretch the trunk up. Stay for 30–60 seconds, then repeat on the other side.

Stand in Tadasana (no. 1), facing the wall. Raise the right foot on to a stool. Straighten both the legs. Hold the belt with the left hand, place the right hand on the right hip and turn the trunk to the right. Stay for 20–30 seconds, then repeat on the other side.

SARVANGASANA (ON WALL)
NECK BALANCE ON WALL

Do Sarvangasana against a wall (no. 38). Stay for 3–5 minutes, then bend the legs and come down.

BHARADVAJASANA
SIMPLE TWIST

Do Bharadvajasana (no. 33) with the hands against a wall to help you twist. Stay for 20–30 seconds, then repeat on the other side.

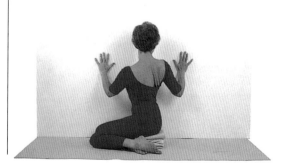

SUPTA PADANGUSTHASANA

RECLINING FINGER-TO-FOOT POSE

All three variants should be practised.

LEG UP

Lie near a column or door post. Bend the left leg and take it up against the post, at 90° to the ground. Support the whole leg, from the buttock to the heel. Extend the right leg along the floor. Stay for 30–60 seconds, then repeat on the other side.

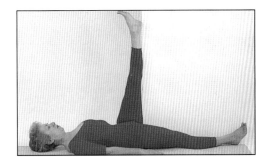

LEG SIDEWAYS

Lie on the floor with the feet against a wall. Bend the left leg over the abdomen and place a belt around the foot. Raise and straighten the leg, then turn it outward in its socket and take it down to the left. Rest the foot on a block or pile of books. Stay for 30–60 seconds, then repeat on the other side.

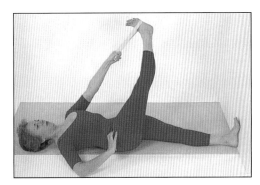

LEG ACROSS

Lie on the floor with the feet against a wall. Bend the right leg, put a belt round the foot and hold it. Straighten the leg, then hold the belt with the left hand and take the leg sideways down to the left. Do not let the left leg turn inward. Stay for 30–60 seconds, then repeat on the other side.

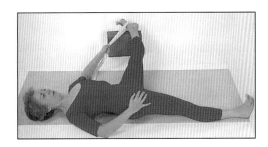

SAVASANA

CORPSE POSE

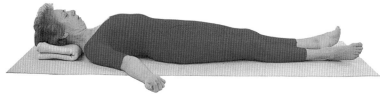

Do Savasana (no. 41). Stay for 5–10 minutes, then turn to the side and get up.

NAMES OF THE POSTURES

Yoga postures are all named in Sanskrit, the classical language of India. In the Asanas section, an English equivalent has been given, either in a direct translation or a description.

The names have been transliterated according to international convention, but omitting the relevant diacritical marks. However, to help readers who wish to learn the correct pronunciation, the postures and other Sanskrit words that appear in the text are listed here with their diacritical marks.

The following points should be noted:

Stress: This is usually on the first syllable. The ā of āsana is always stressed.

Vowels: Long vowels are indicated by a bar over the letter.

Consonants:
c is pronounced "ch".
ś and ṣ are pronounced "sh".
h following any consonant (kh, gh, ph, bh, ch) should be pronounced

distinctly to differentiate it from unaspirated consonants.

ṭ, ḍ, ṇ, are pronounced retroflexively (with the tongue curled back).

ṛ is a semivowel, pronounced as a combination of r and i.

ṅ precedes k or g.

ñ precedes c or j.

A more complete guide to pronunciation can be found in *Light on Yoga* and *Yoga: The Iyengar Way* (see Further Reading).

Adho Mukha Śvānāsana	Marīcyāsana I	Siddhasana	Utthita Hasta
Ardha Halāsana	Matsyāsana	Sukhāsana	Pādāṅguṣṭhāsana
Bhāradvājāsana	Pādāṅguṣṭhāsana	Supta Baddhakoṇāsana	Utthita Pārśvakoṇāsana
Daṇḍāsana	Pārśvottānāsana	Supta Vīrāsana	Utthita Trikoṇāsana
Garuḍāsana	Parvatāsana	Tāḍāsana	Viparīta Karaṇī
Gomukhāsana	Paścimottānāsana	Triaṅg Mukhaikapāda	Vīrabhadrāsana I
Halāsana	Prāsarita Pādottānāsana	Paścimottānāsana	Vīrabhadrāsana II
Janusīrṣāsana	Sarvāṅgāsana	Ūrdhva Prasārita Pādāsana	Vīrāsana
Mālāsana	Śavāsana	Utkaṭāsana	Vṛkṣasana
Marīcyāsana	Setu Bandha Sarvāṅgāsana	Uttānāsana	

FURTHER READING

B. K. S. Iyengar, *Light on Yoga*. Harper Collins, 1966

Light on Pranayama, Harper Collins, 1981

The Illustrated Light on Yoga (formerly *The Concise Light on Yoga*), Harper Collins, 1980

Light on the Yoga Sutras of Patanjali, Harper Collins, 1993

The Tree of Yoga, Fine Line Books, 1988

Geeta S. Iyengar, *Yoga: A Gem for Women*, Allied Publishers, 1983

Silva, Mira and Shyam Mehta, *Yoga: The Iyengar Way*, Dorling Kindersley, 1990

The Upanisads (any edition)

The Bhagavad Gita (any edition)

USEFUL ADDRESSES

Contact the centres listed for information about local Institutes.

UK

Iyengar Yoga Institute
223A Randolph Avenue
London W9 1NL

Manchester & District Institute of Iyengar Yoga
134 King Street
Dukinfield
Tameside
Greater Manchester

Edinburgh Iyengar Yoga Centre
195 Bruntsfield Place
Edinburgh EH10 4DQ

US

BKS Iyengar Yoga National Association of the United States, Incorporated
8223 W. Third Street
Los Angeles
CA 90038

Iyengar Yoga Association of Northern California
2404 27th Avenue
San Francisco
CA 94116

Iyengar Yoga Institute of New York
27 W. 24th Street
Suite 800
New York
NY 10011

Iyengar Yoga Association of Massachusetts, Inc.
240-A Elm Street
Somerville
MA 02114

Iyengar Yoga Association of Minnesota
Box 10381
Minneapolis
MN 55458-3381

Iyengar Yoga Association of Wisconsin
Route 2
Box 70E
La Crosse
WI 54601

Iyengar Yoga Association of the Midwest Bioregions
310 Gralake
Ann Arbor
MI 48103

CANADA

BKS Iyengar Yoga Association
27-F Meadowlark Village
Edmonton
Alberta
T5R 5X4

Centre de Yoga Iyengar de Montreal
919 Mont-Royal Oest
Montreal
PQ H2J 1X3

BKS Iyengar Yoga Association
PO 65694, Station F
Vancouver, BC
V4N 5K7

BKS Iyengar Yoga Association of Ontario
c/o 85 Glenforest Road
Toronto
Ontario
M4N 2A1

AUSTRALIA

BKS Iyengar Association of Australasia
1 Rickman Avenue
Mosman 2088
N.S.W.

Bondi Junction School of Yoga
First Floor
2A Waverly Street
Bondi Junction
Sydney 202
N.S.W.

INDIA

R.I.M. Yoga Institute
1107 B/1 Shivajinagar
Pune 411 016

SOUTH AFRICA

BKS Iyengar Institute
58 Trelawney Road
Pietermaritzburg
Natal 3201

Iyengar Yoga Association of S. Africa
PO Box 78648
Sandton 2146

INDEX

NOTES

NOTES

NOTES

NOTES

NOTES

NOTES

NOTES

NOTES